New Walk

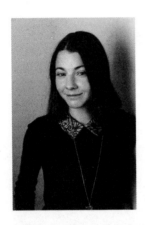

ABOUT THE AUTHOR

Ellie Durant qualified as a midwife in 2010 and worked clinically in the UK and New Zealand. Since 2015 she has been supporting midwives and aspiring midwives with online resources. She is the founder of the 20,000 members strong *Secret Community for Midwives in the Making* and is the author of the bestselling guide for getting into midwifery, *Becoming a Student Midwife: The Survival Guide for Passionate Applicants*. Ellie's blog *Midwife Diaries* is one of the most popular midwifery sites globally. *New Walk* is her first novel.

New Walk

ELLIE DURANT

New Walk (The Midwife Diaries)

First published in Great Britain in 2018 by Pinter & Martin

Copyright © Ellie Durant 2018

All rights reserved.

ISBN 978-1-78066-470-5

Also available as ebook

The right of Ellie Durant to be identified as the author of this work has been asserted by her in accordance with the Copyright, Designs and Patents Act of 1988.

A CIP catalogue record for this book is available from the British Library.

Cover design: Blok Graphic, London
Cover image: Shutterstock (top and back), Blok Graphic (bottom)

Set in Dante

Printed and bound in the EU by Hussar

This book has been printed on paper that is sourced and harvested from sustainable forests and is FSC accredited.

Pinter & Martin Ltd
6 Effra Parade
London SW2 1PS

www.pinterandmartin.com

This book is for Emily Anderson and Jo Stutchbury, a midwife and a doctor who have never met but have a lot in common. Also Pippa. You know why, don't have to say it.

It's also for all student midwives and midwives worldwide. Total heroes.

Author's note
Names, characters, organisations, places, events and incidents are either products of the author's imagination or, in the case of real hospitals and birth centres used as locations, are used fictitiously.

Acknowledgements
Thanks to Kelly Williams, midwife, Steve Topley, paramedic, and Jenna Killett, neonatal nurse, for your professional advice. Thanks Phoenix Writers for everything.

Contents

Prologue

It's my choice. I have a deep sense of rightness about that. I'm glad to be in a country where I can make this choice and I'm glad all the physical stuff, the pain and bleeding and everything at the end, was here at home. Despite the sadness, a bit of me is standing back and assessing the experience for anything that might be useful. I have a kind of morbid curiosity about the emotions and sensations.

This is not the kind of learning anyone would ever want to hear about, though. Even if a woman you were caring for had gone through the same thing, you could never tell her. God forbid you raised your hand in a lecture and talked about it in front of the cohort either.

It's an hour or so before sunset and the temperature is dropping, which I'm grateful for because digging is taking a bit of effort, the earth is dry and set and I'm sore. Despite everything being neglected, the garden is bright with the daisies and red asters that Mum planted. They come up year after year. The birds are talking to each other in different calls and my emotions are blowing around like the breeze.

I'm also thinking about how judgemental I can be. Even

when Dad is hiding from me because he's rolling his tenth spliff of the day and I want to wash his bodywarmer and feed him a healthy tea with green vegetables, or Ali is stalking around in Leicester in heels and and an almost entirely theoretical miniskirt, they are surviving in their own ways.

I put my everything into this life. For years now I've been the passionate, responsible one, reading up on embryology in Mum's old books, studying *Spiritual Midwifery* birth stories over and over until the cover came off, taking every opportunity to learn skills like blood pressure and resuscitation and how to listen. Midwifery is my distraction of choice and I'm proud of that.

But it's also my obsession and underneath I'm not sure I'm coping. I get so angry sometimes. I got so busy lording it over my Dad and my sister that I've found myself here.

I lean the spade against the fence. Before I put the box into the ground I apologise out loud, standing there in my welly boots, which I've put on to dig the hole. I'm truly, deeply sorry.

I'm beginning to understand now. I'm not in control of life; no one is. It never turns out the way you expect. You just make the best of things. This is not always a bad thing; it's just a true thing.

It's both the magic and the catch.

1

Family

Sunday, 12th December 1999

I'm walking home from the Royal Infirmary after a shift and the cold is biting through my gloves. I'm late off and the sun is sending the last few drops of orange light over a frozen dusting of snow on the pavement.

Mum used to tell us about one winter when the snow was eight foot deep. I suspect what she actually meant was eight foot up against the walls, not on the flat, but still, loads more snow than we get today, all over the country, not just in Leicester.

She was five years old and the kids from the old red-brick gasworks houses had a *National Geographic* on Eskimos. They copied the photos, packing and cutting snow into bricks and building an igloo. They even had a window made of ice that they'd taken from the frozen-over canal.

Funny how these stories pop into my head as I walk around Leicester, depending on the weather. They sort of wait for me on street corners and mug me.

The cold is bringing me back to the present. I turn left onto Lincoln Street and, as it's Saturday, the Highfields kids are still out feuding and shouting and getting soaked from snowballs.

A patient died in the night so we were going at warp speed as soon as the shift started, no time to get the breakfast trolley. The shift was important because I learnt to lay a dead person out. Professionally, I mean. The first person I did that for was Mum.

I'm not sure the matron wanted me to learn after-death care. I heard her at the desk saying, *'She's only eighteen!'* But the healthcare assistants know all about Mum and my career plans. They know I can handle it. The woman we laid out looked ready to go, but Mum didn't look like that, she just looked like herself rather than a dead person. I saw her a few hours after she'd died. It was only later that it began to occur to me that it was real, but it helped to be able to wash her and do her nails and make-up. Ali came in to see her when I'd finished and Dad didn't want to wash her either, so I guess they will remember her differently to me. I'm glad I saw the changes. Later in the funeral home we put flowers in her hair and that helped too.

As I go up the steps and put my key in the lock I think about how caring for a dead woman is so much easier than looking after someone with dementia. It's terrible, I know. I have so much patience for anyone having a baby, but I'm not sure I have the right temperament for elderly work. When we'd finished washing and dressing our patient, combing her hair and propping her on the pillows, we felt we'd done well for her. How can you feel that way if you're caring for someone who's always upset and confused? The dead woman looked asleep when her daughter and son arrived and I went back to doing the tea round.

In the hall, I'm greeted by the smell of Dad having smoked himself into a stupor all afternoon. He's on his hands and knees with his head stuck in the cupboard. The hall is full of unfurling carrier bags, little-known bits of the hoover and other under-the-stairs items, and there's an insistent beeping coming from somewhere.

He pulls his head out and says hello without looking at me and then goes back to searching. He's got red-rimmed eyes.

'Hello? Dad?'

'Smoke alarm,' he mutters, 'took the batteries out but it's still going. Fucksake.'

I force myself not to lecture him. He can't have taken the batteries out if it's still beeping. Far more likely is he took it down when it started to make the noise, wrapped it in carrier bags and hid it at the back of the cupboard, hoping the problem would disappear.

'D'you want a hand?'

'Nah, you're okay. Busy shift was it?'

'Not bad.'

I worry about him being on his own all day. I'm out all week with college and then I have a healthcare assistant shift either Friday evening or Saturday on the elderly ward and then antenatal class on Sundays.

He's stopped working. I know he's grieving. But catching him at it is like one of those Attenborough documentaries where you wait for the mountain lions to come out. You only know they've been there because of the paw-prints and the odd carcass strewn around. With Dad this means torn up bits of roach and tobacco sprinkled everywhere.

'Did you do the spuds?'

'What? Yeah. Oh, I mean no.' He's still pulling things out of the cupboard. 'Ali's not coming. She's teaching a class.'

'What class?'

'I dunno, hip-hop or something.'

'Oh, ok.' I try and keep the disappointment out of my voice.

'It's good she's got the work, isn't it?'

'Guess so.'

I leave Dad to it and go and put the kettle on and poke the chicken. I got up at the crack of five forty-five to start it off. It's not just any chicken, it has red peppercorns and white wine, a family recipe. It's really easy. He needed easy things when he and Mum were both working full time. He's a really good cook, he's got scrapbooks full of recipes pasted from magazines and newspapers. But since Mum died he hasn't made much more than toast.

Helga, our big lady tabby cat, knows the sound of the crockpot lid on the kitchen side and turns up to rub herself on my legs and make low, outraged yowling noises.

'Isn't meant for you, though, is it?...'

I pull off a bit of chicken breast and blow on it to cool it down before giving it to her, because she gulps things whole.

I take my tea up to my room. As I go and take my uniform off, before I get in the shower I catch sight of my pale self in the mirror and have to laugh. *Christ girl, is that your happy-to-be-home face?*

The water is almost too hot to stand but feels heavenly on my still-cold skin. I warm up my hands and feet and think about talking to Dad about the weed thing. The grip seal bags are everywhere – in the washing basket, down the sofa – and they always have bits of bud left in them. It's going to be really hard to explain if I accidentally take one to work and someone sees.

I just don't know what to think about it. There's nothing in my textbooks or midwifery books about weed. I have one library book called *Marijuana: The Facts,* which has taught me nothing. It's just a dimmer switch for your brain, the opposite of coffee. You're not supposed to be able to get addicted to it.

I quickly blow-dry my hair and put on my jeans, a vest, two jumpers and my slippers because it's freezing and, though I love our Victorian house with all its mosaic tiling and high ceilings, it's almost impossible to heat it.

I can hear some of Dad's pothead mates have come round and are smoking with him in the living room like we agreed wouldn't happen. Black Sabbath is blasting through the closed door. The smoke alarm by this point is near hysterical, so I find it easily enough, stuffed inside a bicycle pannier, and I tidy everything in the hall away.

I'm about to join whoever's in the lounge, probably Roger by the sound of things, when I hear a voice I don't know say, 'Ayahuasca, that's the shit. DMT y'know man. Tony Blair should smoke it. It's the drug they take to trip balls and seek truth in the jungle, it should be every politician's sacred prescription...'

I laugh so hard I nearly spill my tea and go back upstairs.

I have my UCAS statements to finish; I want all the applications sent by Christmas. I'm applying up North mostly. The midwifery course in Liverpool is supposed to be amazing and the city looks really cool. Of course, it'll be a wrench to leave, but maybe I can do long-distance with Christopher.

Helga comes and sits on my bed and stares at me.

'Don't look at me like that. Dad can feed you. I'll take you to Nanna's if he can't.' She seems ok with that and starts licking and I start writing.

I'm in my flow on holistic care and my experience supporting midwives at the antenatal class when I hear the door slam. By the force of the noise, I know it's Ali. I brace myself for distraction and she bounds up the stairs and hugs me from behind, kissing the top of my head.

She smells like cold air and musky community centre and plasticky body spray over the top.

'Hey,' I say, 'God, you're freezing. Are you wet through?'

'We've been having a snowball fight, it was great!' She roots through my drawer and pulls out my pyjamas, strips naked, her boobs bouncing in the mirror. She throws her wet clothes on the carpet and I pointedly pick them up and put them in my washing basket, but she ignores me.

'Have you been shut up here all day?'

'No. I had a shift.'

She flops onto the bed, grabbing Helga, who mewls a bit as she was sleeping. She knows by now there's no use fighting my big sister.

'How was your class?'

'Great, totally amazing. It's all about the music choice. *Spice Girls* and *Destiny's Child* all the way. Proper little money spinner.'

'The *Spice Girls*? Really?'

'Yeah, I mean, we're playing it ironically. But the mums love it. On the millennium we're going to do a striptease and then head to the Lizard Lounge. You should come, I'll get you in for free.'

'I only ever understand about ten per cent of what you say. What's going on? You and your class are all going to get naked and head out for the millennium? Wouldn't you get arrested?'

'Oh God no, that'd be gross. All those single mums grinding away on the pole... more like your job... did I mention we had a pole? They bring PJs to take off but they have hot pants and stuff on underneath.'

'Mmm, ok, tempting. I'll think about it. Dad said this class you taught tonight was last-minute or something?'

'Yeah, kind of,' she says, looking in the mirror, not meeting my eye.

'Are you going to be around for Christmas?'

'Maybe. Not sure yet.'

She's all twenty-two and curly red hair and curves and she's enjoying herself too much to be bothered with us.

I look at her properly. She has pupils like saucers.

'Ali. Is that not illegal?'

'What?'

'I'm not stupid.'

'Oh God, Chlo, no one cares as long as we turn up and teach a good class. This is just left over from last night anyway. Got a freebie.'

'Who's this guy?'

'You don't know him. He's a terrific shag though. I mean, when he's not on e.'

'I hope you're being safe.'

I regret saying this as soon as the words are out of my mouth. Ali's like a freight train when she's taken ecstasy, she'll do and say anything, faster than you can keep up with. It's not a time to argue. Helga's purring is getting louder as Ali is fussing her more.

'You're so serious, aren't you? Have a bit of fun Chloe. Speaking of which, how's Christopher? He's a patient guy, isn't he?'

Christopher is not a fan of Ali's, though she doesn't know this. He thinks she's irresponsible and I take on too many of her problems. I turn back and start writing again, hoping she'll get the idea and leave.

'What are you doing, homework? Oh. Nice. Uni admissions. Off to be a midwife?'

There are reasons why that question stings. Growing up I

thought an older sister might be a helpful thing, that I'd always have someone to turn to, apart from Mum. Then I realised that each time I did talk to her I'd come away confused and hating myself. I don't know how she does it. She looks over my shoulder.

'Maybe.'

'Who's going to look after Dad? And Helga?'

'Can we not talk about this now? *Please?*'

She shakes her head.

'I'm just asking. I'm not saying it should be you. We should just talk about this stuff.'

I lose it. A snapping, snarling corkscrew of anger escapes.

'I *always* want to talk about this stuff. But I hate working this hard and planning dinner around you two and trying to make sure it happens and keeping us together. Neither of you cares. So yes, I am thinking about moving away. I'm the only one putting any effort in.'

She looks at me with her wide black pupils.

'*Jesus.* Get off your high horse.'

Then she dumps Helga on the bed and slams my door.

I breathe and look out at the evening. There are tiny crystals of ice floating in the spectrum of the streetlights, dancing, pushed by the wind. I hear her downstairs saying,

'Dad, splash round your ciggies.'

I copy out the last few lines of my statement. I have one last choice to make. It's between Plymouth and here. From Plymouth you can travel, it has ferries, my time off could be filled with France, Italy, Spain or even further. I'd moonlight as a healthcare assistant for a year if it meant I could go to Africa.

I can hear Dad downstairs banging on, something about converting the attic being a good project for his carpentry skills, as if he'll ever get round to that. And then how Egyptians smoked weed, definitely, and they started civilisation.

I sigh. It's not like Leicester Uni is bad. Mum trained here.

When I've finished and I go downstairs it's nearly midnight. Ali looks tired now, the drugs must be wearing off. She's watching *Friends* with the sound turned down.

She looks up at me and stretches her arms out and I relax into her familiar embrace. I haven't forgiven her, but I do miss her.

We sit in the dark for a long time and she strokes my hair. I think we're both taking in Dad slumped on the sofa, looking about ten years older than he actually is, unshaven and in a shirt covered with holes where he's dropped tiny bits of burning tobacco and weed.

'I'm hungry,' I say eventually. We make sandwiches from the chicken and eat them in the dining room, the hot stock and fat dripping into the white sliced bread. Ali falls asleep on the sofa and I go to bed soon after. I've got college in the morning.

2

Christopher

We've set off from Jos's and are winding our way through town, past the clock tower, neon-lit takeaways, boarded-up jewellers' shops and student digs with the lights off. The guys are jumping over bollards like monkeys and the girls are chatting. I'm out with the Regent's College crowd, on the way to a death metal gig at the Princess Charlotte.

I'm tense. Christopher may not turn up to a band called 'Eerily Murdered', but then again he might, and then try and take me away to somewhere more tasteful, which would be a pain because I want to enjoy this. We'll all be heading our separate ways to uni in six months.

As me and Jos avoid broken glass and vomit on the pavement (the Charlotte is not a venue for heels, so we've opted for trainers) I can see she's watching Hamza.

I reach for her hand and squeeze it. 'He's not going anywhere,' I say. I'm thinking of Christopher and the possibility of leaving. There's an intense centre-of-the-universe feeling he gives me that I'm beginning to suffer without, and it's only been a week since I last saw him.

She sighs, 'Thanks. I wish he was though. Then I could follow him.'

'I thought he was going to Brighton? To do physics? Or maths was it?'

'If he can concentrate hard enough on his A-levels it'll be maths. But his *Ammi* wants him to stay here now.'

'You're kidding.'

'Nope. She's going to get him a wife, big wedding, all that. If he's living at home, it's harder for him to see me.'

'Bugger.'

'Yeah. I go around there and his Mum can't wait to make the point over and over, *oh it's Hamza's good friend, just like his sister.*'

'Yeah. You're lucky to have found each other, I just wish they could see it.'

As we watch, Hamza rugby tackles one of his friends and they both fall over shouting and he looks back at Jos to check she's seen. She looks at him in a way that's more parental than anything else and I can't help but smile.

'You'd think I'd be exactly what they wanted. I've been keeping him out of trouble for years now, getting him to study, stopping him eating bacon butties. I know more about Islam than his Mum at this point. It's not my fault my family's not from Pakistan! I would have loved to grow up Muslim.'

This all comes out in a torrent and I feel bad. I've been neglecting her for revision, Dad, shiftwork and Christopher.

Jos was the one person to get what we were going through when Mum died. She made me feel normal. If I'm really honest with myself, I might have been avoiding her. It's hard, the Islam thing, like she's tuned into a different frequency and the volume's slowly being turned up.

We queue and are ticketed and ID-ed, which still makes

a refreshing change from breaking in through the toilet windows. I'm not sure we'd get Jos in anyway with her new tendency towards long skirts.

The music is obscenely loud and slams me in the chest as we go in, vibrating my bones. The floor is tiny and near capacity, with the usual mix of metal-heads, the mentally ill and students balancing things out. The warm-up act are playing and there's nothing going on behind their eyes, but Hamza immediately makes his way to the floor and starts headbanging. You can basically see the air in here: it smells of stale beer and men who rarely shower, but dance topless anyway.

Jos squeezes my hand and yells, 'TOILETS' into my ear and Mia and I follow her. It's wet and dirty and the porcelain sinks are thumping with bass, but I can at least hear her.

'Enough about me, I haven't asked if you've heard back from unis yet. What's going on?'

'Oh God, no, don't ask. Nothing so far. Sarah in our year has got her nursing interviews, hasn't she?'

'Maybe midwifery's different, sorting through applications in smaller departments or something though. Don't worry Chloe, it'll happen. They'd be mental not to offer you a place.'

'Maybe. Hey, what's Hamza doing in all of this? Can't he just tell his parents to get stuffed?'

'He's not brave enough.'

'I'd be furious,' I say.

Jos leans on the sink. 'What would be the point in getting angry though? It wouldn't change anything. He's an idiot, but he's my idiot. And he's supposed to respect what they want.'

'He's a hot idiot,' says Mia, over the toilet door, pissing.

It's true. Hamza is a wisp of a nineteen-year-old, with

thick, doe-like black eyelashes contrasting with his rapid energy. He's always wired.

'But it's weird 'cause we all grew up together,' Mia continues, 'It feels like fancying your brother. I shag people I *don't* know.'

Jos ignores this. Mia is a good mate, but she has no filter and started drinking much earlier in the evening.

'I know this sounds melodramatic, but I honestly think if he marries someone else, I'll be heartbroken for the rest of my life. And he helped me find Islam.'

'He loves you.'

'Yeah. But I get where his mum's coming from. Having Muslim kids in this country. All that harassment for your family. They don't want someone white for him, but honestly, I'm not what they think.'

I can feel the thud of the bass coming through the wall I'm leaning on and some kind of sampled organ-music-cum-female-opera layered over the top.

'That's awful,' she says and we start laughing.

'Now you know why his family don't want him to study music at uni. It's a totally un-Islamic choice. If we can just get him through college, he'll grow out of it, but I wish they'd listen to me and get him a tutor. He's fine studying if there's someone sat there with him...'

Mia flushes the toilet and interrupts. 'Is that blonde guy out tonight? 'Manther', is that what they call him? He's fucking cute.'

'Who? What?' I ask.

'She means Chris, I'm afraid,' says Jos and then, 'That's really classy, Mia; back off, he's Chloe's.'

'What did you call him?' I ask, confused.

'Oh, is that Chloe's boyfriend then?'

'Yeah. I wish you wouldn't call him Manther. If he hears it'll make him uncomfortable,' says Jos.

'Is Manther not his name? Thought it was one of those Dutch-type names, long blond hair and all. He answers to that, though, doesn't he?' says Mia, splashing her hands.

Jos frowns and says, 'If he does it's because you're drunk and he's humouring you. Watch yourself.'

Mia shrugs.

'He's not Dutch,' Jos goes on, 'He's from Cambridge, that's where his accent's from. It's just a name Steve came up with. Like a cougar, but male. Male panther. And it kind of caught on...'

Jos catches my expression and adds 'Not that he's that much older! He's great Chloe, we all really like him.'

'How old *is* he?' asks Mia.

'Twenty-five,' says Jos. I wish this wasn't public knowledge. It isn't anyone's business, and an age gap isn't so unusual. We met at one of the evening physiology lectures at Leicester Uni. I was going to go along with Jos. It was on brain development and she's doing psychology so I thought she'd find it useful, and I wanted to go because our biology teacher isn't all that. But Jos dropped out last-minute to go and help Hamza with an essay and I ended up going on my own. Christopher was there helping out and when he smiled at me I lost my mind. Then I saw him out in the Charlotte and said hi and eventually he asked me out.

'Twenty-five. Huh. He's breaking the seven-year law then.'

'What?' I ask.

'If you're shagging someone younger, you can only do it if they're half your age plus seven years or more, otherwise it's illegal.'

Jos wrinkles her nose.

'If you're both adults, there aren't any laws about that kind of thing, I'm pretty sure.'

'Oh,' says Mia, wiping her hands on her skirt, 'Good to know.'

'Plus, Chloe hasn't had sex with him. Have you Chloe?'

I sigh. Everyone is so interested.

'What? He'll think you're a lesbo Chloe, get on with it. You can't just leave a guy waiting for that long, you'll lose him, that's my advice.'

'This is none of your business,' I say in a sing-song voice.

'Whatever. I'm getting a drink.' She slams the door behind her.

'Always the charmer...' says Jos. And then she asks, '*Is* Chris coming tonight?'

'Christopher. He gets annoyed if you call him Chris. And he'll like 'Manther' even less. It's a stupid name, I really hope he doesn't ever hear it, it'd be terrible to have to explain... Hey, what was that word you used? A revert?' She'll know I'm trying to distract her, but she'll take the opportunity to talk, she needs to.

'Everyone is born knowing Allah. If you're not born into an Islamic family, you can get things wrong to begin with. And then you can do your Shahada like me and revert to God. They do all these courses at the mosque.'

A goth girl with a nose ring and spikes round her neck comes in and gets out a substantial makeup bag, giving Jos a really weird look in the mirror.

'I see. Hey, I'm glad you're happy. It makes sense for you.'

'I'm not trying to force it on anyone, it's just so comforting. Learning Arabic especially, it's a beautiful language. It's hard but worth it, it means you can read the Q'uran properly.'

'Yeah. I know. Just do what you think is best. I will too. We'll both end up happy, *Inshallah*' I say, God willing. That brings this conversation arc to an end, as I'm not sure I like where it's headed. I love Jos but there's no way I'm adding Arabic and Islamic studies to my workload.

'*Inshallah,*' she says. There's some applause as the first band finish and some backing music comes on.

'*Are* you going to sleep with him?' She asks it fast, trying to draw me out by surprising me, in front of someone we don't know, like that's going to work. I'm not sure whether this is vicarious living or she's interested, or worried.

I just smile. I'm irritated but I take her hand and we go and join the girls from my biology class who've staked out their bit of the crammed mosh pit. The real band are coming on.

We all scream as the vocalist, a towering skeleton in a red silk shirt, sets himself up and the drummer starts abusing his kit. The first phenomenally loud chords shake us and we dance, alternately sticking to the floor and slipping on something that's best not investigated. But soon I forget about this and my arms are in the air. The band knows how to whip things up and it's a frenzy. Jos and I are dancing together to fend off the crowd. This little Leicester group of us, we're moving together like a wave, jumping up and down like we've got our own gravity. I get lost in thoughts and dreams and hot hope in my stomach.

Then someone pinches me on the bum, hard and I turn around to slap whoever it is, but it's just Ali, laughing. She's all in black, not enough material covering her porcelain white body, and she screams 'SPOOKY MUSIC!' Her pupils are massive. Again.

'DON'T DRINK TOO MUCH!' I try and scream, but she can't hear. She's in raptures to be in here and I can't help feeling a bit proud of the way she can move. She's gathering attention, people are watching her.

We go on like this for a few songs and then I get pissed off by being elbowed in the ear by one of the biology girls who has her tongue down the throat of some sound guy they call Feedback Phil. This is a pretty gross thing to be watching so I strategise my way out of the crowd and there he is. Christopher, in a suede jacket and pale blue shirt, shouting what he wants across the bar.

Then he sees me and smiles. I have a small moment of stillness in which I can stand back and see how much trouble I'm in. His thin cheeks remind me of cliffs. He pulls me over, kissing me on the cheek and clamping me under one arm.

I breathe him in. I think he's fresh from a shower.

From here I can see Ali being whirled around on someone's shoulders, which looks dangerous among so many bodies. Sure enough, that area of the floor explodes into a fight. She's caught someone's face with her Doc Martens and there's a guy yelling at her and pinching his nose, which is bleeding. I don't think Christopher has seen so I shout in his ear, 'Good day?' to distract him.

He starts shouting in reply and waving his hand around. I can't hear, but I nod anyway, looking over his shoulder to see what's happening to Ali.

When I look back the bouncers have got involved and hauled the guy off. Ali's got away scot free, just standing there with her hands on her hips, screaming, and Jos's mouth is open, a few spots of blood on her white shirt.

Christopher follows my gaze and frowns. I see rather than hear him say 'Oh, for God's sake.'

'I'm really sorry,' I say and I get up to go and sort things out, but he doesn't drop my hand so I sort of ricochet back to him. He shakes his head, 'No.'

'I should just go and check...'

'No. Come on, let's go.' He leaves his half-drunk beer on the bar and grabs my hand.

I can see Jos and Hamza calming Ali down and getting her back into the mosh pit. Christopher is leaning over the coat room counter and pointing out my jacket and I pass over my ticket and struggle into it and my scarf as fast as I can. His expression is grim.

I follow him out into the night with a sinking heart.

'Are you okay?'

He doesn't answer. It's got much colder since we've been inside; my dress is sleeveless and my jacket isn't thick enough to keep out the wind. I'm struggling to keep up as we pass a guy with a paper cup of change, his small, sad Jack Russell curled up with him under a blue sleeping bag. The cold is already making it hard for me to think, so God knows how the homeless guy feels.

Christopher is still not saying anything. We walk over the ring road, past the arch of the old city stones, which contrast so strangely with the clubs and pubs, and cross to the university campus, where the ivy-covered buildings are all lit up in the moonlight. Within minutes I'm shivering so badly that my stomach muscles are aching. I just want him to say something.

He's squeezing my hand, his steps echoing off the pavement.

'Where are we going?'

'Back to mine.'

'Oh. Okay.'

It's horrible that the first time we'll go back to his it will be in the middle of a fight. Or is this a fight?

I want to stop him and insist on hearing what's going on,

but I think digging my heels in is the immature thing to do. And it's freezing. We're walking towards the bridge, Narborough Road way. The smell of fried onions and spice from the Indian takeaways is making me a bit hungry and a bit sick. I knew he lived in this direction, but not where exactly and even though I'm tired and cold and worried, I'm also curious.

We turn left into one of the avenues and straight up some concrete steps. At his door, he unlocks three separate bolts and points me in before him, into the warm.

It's open plan and smells like lemon cleaning spray. The navy blue carpets have a freshly hoovered air and a cafetière and blender are all that's out on the kitchen side. A wok hangs on the wall. Christopher exhales.

My fingers are numb, the nails stinging from the blood coming back into them. I want to run to the radiator to warm my hands, chilblains be damned, but I stand uncertainly, the noise of the Charlotte still ringing in my ears.

'Should I take my shoes off?'

'Yeah. Please. It's my Dad's really, this place, I'm renting it from him. Well I mean, it's in my name, but it's a loan,' he says, 'Are you having a drink? Wine, whisky?'

I don't like either and I wish I could ask for tea but I say, 'Whatever you're having is fine.'

I watch him fumble around in a drawer.

'This is a really nice Sauvignon. I'll get some glasses... go and have a look around if you like, do the tour,' he waves a corkscrew towards the stairs.

I slip my trainers off and leave them on the mat and pad up in my tights, feeling weird, like I'm snooping. But it's a good distraction. My heart is fluttering like a trapped bird and I'm relieved he doesn't seem angry now he's home.

The spare room is tiny and empty and the door hits the bed

as I open it as there's so little space. Clearly no one sleeps here. The bathroom is also spartan, blue tiles and a yellow towelling dressing gown hanging up. I run my hands under the hot tap and they start to warm, painfully. In the shaving mirror I'm a pale girl in a sensible black dress, with heavy eyebrows and a small chest. The same.

In Christopher's room, across the hall, an outsize spherical lamp shade is catching the air current from the window and swaying. It's a large room with a double bed and thin windows that rattle as cars go past. There's a cactus on the windowsill that makes monstrous shadows on the blinds.

'Chloe?'

'Coming...'

I go back downstairs and Christopher smiles and hands me a glass of white wine and we sit together on the leather sofa. The warmth is making me relax and I breathe and summon up my courage.

'So. Why are you annoyed with me?'

'What? I'm not,' he looks at me and I take in his eyes, steel-blue contrasting with his dark eyelashes. 'What makes you think I'm annoyed?'

'Hurrying out of the Charlotte like that.'

'How's the wine?'

I take a big gulp. It tastes like paint stripper.

'It's great. I'm sorry, I didn't mean to spoil your evening.'

'Oh, you didn't. Not really my scene anyway. You're spending too much time on your sister though. And I don't know what's going on with your Dad, but...'

The few times Christopher has picked me up from mine I think he's seen some of the issues. We haven't commented on Dad much. We stick to safer conversations like study and jobs and travel. Sometimes Ali, but usually not.

'He's had a hard time of it recently.'

'So have you.'

'Yeah, but he's not so good at accepting help.'

'Apart from help from you.'

I'm not really sure what he's trying to say so I take another sip. It burns going down. I try and explain my sister and Dad.

'It's been a rough few years for him. For him and Ali both. They're similar people.'

He takes the glass off me and puts his hand on my face, 'You really are the sweetest girl.'

When he kisses me his lips and tongue are coated with the acrid wine but I don't care. I have a constellation of half panic, half joy in my stomach. He pulls back and looks at me.

'You're going to get three As, right, for your A-levels? And you're on track with care experience?'

'I'll try. Probably a B in chemistry, but that's okay, unis won't be bothered.'

'Have you thought about doing medicine?'

'I haven't – ' I clear my throat, nonplussed, 'I haven't got any interviews for midwifery even.'

'I think we can safely say they'll be interested. But in terms of careers, you'd make an excellent doctor, wouldn't you? Wouldn't that be better? You could do obstetrics if you're set on that side of things.'

I wasn't expecting this. To cover my confusion I ask, 'Did *you* ever want to be a doctor?'

'No. I like research. You're talented with people though, you need to be interacting with them in whatever profession you end up in. You get a bit older and you can see these things. I wish I'd been pushed just a bit further when I was your age and got into Cambridge or Oxford. It's worth being successful early if you can...'

He kisses me again, in a way we haven't kissed before, a long, lingering kiss and my thoughts are jumbled.

I think about how royally annoyed Mum would be to hear him trying to talk me out of midwifery. I think about Ali and whether or not she's been thrown out of the Charlotte and Dad who sometimes leaves the hob on so you come back to a black crusted mass of baked beans at the bottom of a pan and coal black chips because the oven's been on all night.

Christopher's hands go under my dress, grazing the outside of my thighs, and the feeling of his thumbs through my tights is electric. I make a small, involuntary noise and he smiles against my lips.

'Thanks,' I say, 'For the vote of confidence.'

He pulls back for a second and says 'It's up to you. You might want other things in life that won't fit with medicine, midwifery might be better. For a family and so on,' and before I can respond, he pulls me back to him.

A bit of my mind is trying to follow what he said about families and trying the possibility on because *was that a hint?* But it's heavenly, the contours of my body are fitting into his, he's exploring my mouth with his tongue and his hand disappears under my dress again, his fingers in slow circular motion and *oh my God...*

Then he stops and it's almost painful.

'Chloe. Have you done this before?'

'Er. Yes.' He smiles again, pulls me to my feet, hands me my wineglass and starts to lead me up the stairs.

I've answered too fast. My brain is so full that I've misunderstood the question. Yes, I have been touched before at the back of a house party with a boy out of his mind and his hands down my jeans. But not like *this*.

As we go into Christopher's room, he pushes me onto his

bed and rolls me to one side to unzip my dress. I realise this is actually happening and my heart starts thumping.

'D'you want some music on?'

'No, it's okay. Oh, I mean, well if it's no bother, yes.'

He rolls off me and hits a button on the CD player, turning the volume down.

'Do you know who this is?'

'No.'

'It's Prince.'

'Oh, okay. Christopher?'

'Yes?'

'When I said I'd done this before...'

'*Oh.*'

'I'm nervous. It's silly,' I'm croaking, how attractive.

'Hey, we don't have to do this. But if we do, I'll be really gentle. Are you on the pill?'

'Yeah. I started taking it...'

I'm cold again now, in my best pink underwear (thank God I chose to wear it today) and he's fully clothed, which doesn't feel right and his jeans have little metal studs on which dig in. They make me jump when he positions himself above me. Then he relaxes and his weight is spread out and that's better. I breathe against him.

'Are you okay?'

'Yeah. Um.'

'You sure?'

'I have a silly question. A silly request.'

'No, go on?'

'Do you have any candles? I always imagined candles.'

He looks stunned, as if he's never heard of such a thing. But then he gets off me and opens his bottom drawer and takes out a packet of matches. In his bedside drawer, along with some batteries, notebooks and a few condoms, are a packet of tea lights.

'Will these do?'

'Yeah.' He lights them, every one.

I spread the candles on his bookshelf, table, on top of his wardrobe. He takes his clothes off, so casually, and reclines, watching me just in his boxers. The pale expanse of his chest, the slight curve of his stomach and the hair tracking down is lovely in the darkness. Soon the room is full of tiny flames flickering in the draught.

When I've finished, he stretches his hand out to pull me back over onto the bed.

'Okay now?'

'Yeah. Lovely. Pretty.'

'Yes. You are.'

Even though I'm nervous, I have to laugh at this and Christopher smiles back, unembarrassed.

He lies on top of me again, one hand in my hair, the other in my underwear. He pushes me in the stomach and makes me jump. I can feel him smiling against my lips. I look down and he's taken his boxers off and *oh my that's the first time I've seen one of those apart from at work and this is a bit different*. My breath catches in my throat.

When he pushes into me, I feel like the bed is moving, like a boat in the sea and I close my eyes. It's a deep, stretching pain and I grab onto the bed covers with one hand. After a while, I realise the tension is making it worse and I relax. It's better.

When it's over he cups me from behind and pulls my thighs apart. He's well practised at this, but I'm sore and a bit freaked out so it takes me a long time to come. But when I do it's huge, like a wave crashing over me. We lie together as our sweat cools and he hugs me to him.

Almost immediately afterwards, I start to worry about the candles. As if he's in my head, Christopher gets up and blows them all out, the little lights dying one by one. The smoke lingers and makes me think of birthdays.

He comes back to bed and cuddles me again, one arm firmly over me, like a dog with a stick.

The streetlight comes through the curtain and I lie awake in the dark. His body is just the right temperature to keep me warm. But I can't sleep for a long time.

The morning is so sweet. I don't understand how people don't spend their entire lives kissing: in bed, on the stairs, up against the kitchen counter. I haven't even brushed my teeth, I have coffee breath because he made me a cappuccino with his posh machine, but he doesn't seem to care.

We spend a long time talking about his family. His Mum's a researcher and his Dad teaches at a uni. We don't mention mine again.

'Are you okay, then? Are you sure you won't stay for breakfast? Bacon sandwich?'

'No. I need to get back. I've got a night shift and I need to do all the jobs before that.'

I'm at the door and I've borrowed a big blue jumper for the walk home. It still looks freezing out there. I'm turning the cuffs up so they don't dangle. Christopher is sitting on the bottom step of the stairs, in his dressing gown, his hair sticking up in all directions. He looks like a kitten that's had its hair licked.

'Last night was... come here,' he hugs me to him. 'Was it okay for you?'

'It was...' Romantic? Painful? The most human thing I've ever done? 'Wonderful. Important.'

'Is that a good thing?'

'Yes. Thank you.' I kiss him goodbye, trying to put reassurance into it because he looks so uncertain.

When I get home, I find Dad has half burnt one tea towel in the kitchen, apparently while cooking a ham and cheese Findus crispy pancake in a frying pan, and his grinder is on the kitchen table. The lounge has a pile of clean washing in the middle of the floor, fragrantly sprinkled with rolling tobacco. There are some pencil sketches distributed around, of boxes and dimensions, in his practised hand. I'm hoping this means he's got work at last.

When I go upstairs, the loo roll is trapped in the closed bathroom window. It's fluttering in the breeze. This strikes me as hilarious.

'Chloe?'

Dad appears at the loo doorway, gangly and frowning.

'What's happening, what's funny?'

'Nothing at all. How are you?'

'Fine.' He shuffles off back to his room and I follow, wanting to check in there for plates and dirty sheets, but he turns and says, 'You don't need to come in.'

'Um...okay...'

'Thank you,' he says, primly.

'Sure. Bring down your empties.'

I do the Saturday jobs: mop the floors, fold up the washing and put another load on. When it's clean downstairs, I run a bath and shave my legs, pensively, wondering if Christopher noticed the slight stubble. I didn't have time to do them on

Friday. I touch myself, the warm water lapping at the sensitivity and a small trail of blood escapes into the water and disperses.

I choose black underwear and take some paracetamol. I'm tired, sore and headachy and deeply happy and I wrap myself in my dressing gown, longing for a lie down. I want to think about everything, to reflect, to let it all get settled in my memory and to sleep before my night on the elderly ward. I also want to set the dishwasher off, but before I do so I go and knock on Dad's door.

'No! Don't come in.'

He's not usually so touchy. I push the door a crack, 'I'm just after empties. Did you forget?'

I can hear him rummaging around in there. It doesn't smell brilliant, like musty clothes. But then I get a whiff of something else, something potent, and I hover with my fingertips on the handle, considering.

A bit of me would rather not know what he's up to. It's not my business. I'm his daughter not his parent, and I'd like today to be entirely about me for once. Also, I don't think he wants my input and if I don't know what's happening then I don't have to do anything about it.

But any time I haven't followed the clues with Dad, it's always come back at me.

I push the door fast to catch him, feeling only slightly bad about it.

In the dingy light the carpet is scattered with clear polythene bags grouped into different sizes. There's an open wooden joinery box decorated with flat brass diamonds in which sits a silver set of digital scales. Five bunches of dark brown bud, still on the stalk and each as big as my fist, are lined up on the duvet cover.

He's even got a cash box, a red one, and a small notebook

with figures scribbled in it.

He's standing there with a pillow like he can cover some of it up. There's a long silence while I try to find the right words.

He breaks it first.

'It's just a plant, Chloe. Something we've been using for three thousand years or more, it's always been around, traded just like tea or salt...'

'Tea won't get me fired. Or you arrested.'

'Chloe, don't start, or I will... some of the stuff you get round here, it's much better to buy it like this, wholesale... remember, your Mum liked a smoke.'

'Oh, don't try that one, it's beneath you! She joined in with you when she'd had a rubbish day and couldn't be telling you off anymore!'

He's cowering and that makes me feel powerful and then sick at myself. I try to be calm. We can work through this, we can cope with this.

'I thought they asked you to teach at that college?'

No answer.

'Do you have any work at all?'

He's not looking at me, he's staring at the floor.

'Dad? Have you lost your job?'

'No. I haven't.'

He meets my eye now. There's fear in his expression but screw him, I'm furious.

'You know what, I'm so fed up with the way you treat me. I do the washing. I do my shifts. I lend you money. You could make more money teaching carpentry in an hour than I can on a whole shift.'

He's startled now.

'I'm off work.'

'Why?'

'I'm depressed.'

I don't want to talk about it, but I suddenly want him to see it from my point of view.

'You have no idea if you're depressed. You're too high to even work it out. D'you think I don't think about Mum every day?'

His mouth is open and I know I've won already, but now I've started I can't stop.

'And it's not a bad thing, okay? I want to remember her. Of course I feel like she's missing, every moment. I'm eighteen and she's my Mum! But you have to feel it at some point! You can't just sit here smoking for the next twenty years!'

He doesn't respond.

'What do you think Mum would say to you now?'

Again, silence. I think he's angry at the question. Well fuck him, I'm angry at everything. I'm tired of not being answered.

'Get rid of it. Or I'll call the police.'

'You wouldn't.'

'I really would! I'd rather it was the police than you getting beaten up by some gang!'

He has dirty clothes and mugs all over the floor. I can't think what else to do so I start to gather them up. Stacked to one side is a big pile of letters, some of the envelopes ripped up for roach.

'Oh my God, Dad, is this all the post?'

I dig through and there's one from British Gas. I glance at it.

'Have you sorted these? Are we in the red?'

'I'm not a complete fuck-up,' he says quietly. 'I've paid the bills.'

'Why are you hoarding them, then?'

I turn one large envelope over in my hand. It's got my

name on it.

'What's this?' There's another on the floor near it.

'What have you done?'

I don't say anything while I gather up every letter on the floor that's addressed to me and slam his door on my way out.

In my own room, I sit down at my desk. I want to just ignore this; I want to never open them, never have to find out what it means. I hear Dad put music on, he's playing something classical through the wall. I think it's Schubert, something him and Mum used to listen to. He's trying to calm me down, I think, which makes me even angrier.

I rip open the first envelope. It's stamped from Leeds University.

Dear Miss Cawthorne,

Further to your application for Midwifery training, we are pleased to invite you to attend a selection day as follows:

DATE/TIME: Monday, 17th January 2000, at 8.45am

I open the remaining envelopes. Obviously, because life is very cruel, every interview has been and gone. I sit and cry for a while, hating this, hating him and then... I don't hate him. I feel sorry for him, in a mortifying way, and he's still my Dad, even if he's so screwed up that I don't think he'll ever be normal again.

When I go back into his room, he's sitting at the desk in silence, his head in his hands. All the weed and paraphernalia has been cleared away.

I look at him for a long moment. I can't see whether he meant to do this. But it seems likely. I wonder if I've been so absent he couldn't ask me to stay and couldn't bear me going. I could shout some more, but what would it achieve? He'd just slink away, sorry and upset.

'Dad. We can't have this.'

'I know.'

'Then you'll do the right thing? You'll get rid of it all?'

He looks me in the eye, as steady as he ever gets.

'Yes. If it upsets you that much, then I will.' I don't believe him.

I take his plates and mugs downstairs and stack the dishwasher, before starting to get ready for my shift.

3

Parentcraft

Sunday, 20th August 2000

It's a clammy, overcast evening. I have my rain jacket in my bag as I pedal towards Aylestone Road and I'm trying to ignore the black hole in my stomach. All my mates apart from Jos are moving off to uni in a few weeks and I've got my grades and I did pretty well, but I'm staying in Leicester for another year.

This antenatal class is a descendant of the Birth Information Centre, where Mum used to work for a while. I've been coming for a few years now. At its peak, it was a labyrinth of social workers, nurses, physios and others working in ratty council rooms. I remember being bribed to stay quiet with colouring in and cartons of Ribena, reading posters about HIV before I understood what that meant.

These days funding has been cut and it's just in the St Edward's church room, run by whichever community midwife happens to be free. When I've stashed my bike and put out the chairs and leaflets, I help myself to a biscuit. Then I sit pawing at the battered piano for a bit, out of tune notes floating up to the stone ceiling.

Mum used to sing *I Will Survive* here, with tweaked pregnancy and birth lyrics. It was infectious and she got them all joining in. The thing about Mum was she had very little shame.

I stop when the first couples arrive. They're having discussions about car seats, the contents of their hospital bags and a few are complaining about having to do antenatal class somewhere Catholic. They're from different backgrounds; a few with Indian heritage; a beautifully dressed couple from Ethiopia who've been before and a few who look Eastern European.

They have different skin tones but the same swaying walks, balancing their bumps. The Virgin Mary statue looks on from the corner, bored. She's been there and done that already.

The midwife still hasn't arrived by eight so I stand at the front and introduce myself and apologise. There hasn't been a phone call so she's probably on her way. The atmosphere is good now, they're all swapping numbers. And we have lots of custard creams and bourbons to give them after, if nothing else.

As I'm speaking the door opens. Everyone cranes around to see who's arrived late. It's a young girl with bleached blonde hair, a silver ring in her nose and big black headphones around her neck. She's glaring. I give her a little wave.

'Hi. Are you joining us for antenatal group?'

She doesn't answer.

'You'd be very welcome to.'

She looks at me for a second, then about turns and lets the door bang shut behind her.

'Hang on, I'll be back,' I say to the class and follow her.

But the girl has disappeared as I head out into the hall. I only got a quick glimpse, but she looked like she might have been crying, her eyes were puffy under the layer of thick concealer. I wonder whether she's got the wrong date. Maybe she was here for a study group or, you never know, she might have wanted to pray.

Then I hear the sound of painful retching and coughing from down the hall. I follow the noise to the toilets and stand next to the sink. She's in the furthest cubicle.

'Hey? You okay, love?'

It doesn't sound like she's bringing up much, she's just dry heaving, but still, I wouldn't want an audience. I stand uncertainly. The toilets have an ancient blue and white tile pattern, it's like being inside a glacier.

I hear her mutter, 'Fuckin' awful.'

'Can I get you some water?'

'Yeah, please...'

I run to the kitchen and when I get back she's washing her hands and looking miserable.

'You alright now?'

She makes a noise, half fed-up, half laugh.

I catch her face reflected in the mirror. Up close I can see she's been crying for sure, her eyes are red-rimmed.

'Is it morning sickness?'

'Oh, fuck off.'

'Sorry.'

I back up, regretting being so forward. But she's not looking at me and she didn't swear with conviction. Sometimes people say the exact opposite of what they mean.

She considers me. I offer her the glass of water.

'Go slowly,' I advise and she takes it from me and sips it and makes a face.

'You a midwife?'

I sigh inwardly. I can't bring myself to talk about my career aspirations, it's too painful. Instead, I say, 'I don't know why they call it morning sickness, it goes on all day. Are you keeping water down?'

'I can keep Milky Bar down.'

'Okay, well, that's a good start. What's your name?'

She freezes and seems to shrink into her hoody.

'I'm Chloe. I'm a volunteer,' I offer.

There's a long pause and then she says, 'Sadie.'

I ask her if she wants a brew and to my relief, she agrees.

As we go past the hall, I see through the glass door that the midwife has finally arrived. She's in a navy blue uniform with lots of silver badges on the collar, has thickly textured blonde hair and an expression of fatigued annoyance. She's taking the class through the breathing exercise. They all have their eyes closed and are inhaling and exhaling for counts of four.

Sadie mutters, 'Fucking bitch...' and I raise my eyebrows.

She sits on a chair with her messenger bag clutched on her lap and she faffs around with a biscuit packet, picking at the seal with her black varnished nails.

When I've made us both a drink I sit next to her. The steam rises from the cups.

'So... are you from round here? Leicester's home for you?'

'Yeah, over in St Matthew's.'

Ah. There are big tower blocks around there, near the industrial estate. It's rough as.

'*She* did my appointment, her in the hall. I want a c-section and she won't let me have one. Said I should bring my Mum in, like she gets it! I'm more likely to end up being chucked out the flat than anything else...'

'How old are you, if you don't mind me asking?'

She looks wary. 'Seventeen.'

I suspect she's sixteen, if that. If she's fifteen there'll be a child protection issue going on. I wonder why she wasn't sent straight off to the teenage pregnancy midwife.

'We're selling kittens and that was all the midwife was interested in. She just kept telling me not to do the cat litter with my bare hands, um, *hello*, like I'm going to do something that stupid and disgusting anyway, let alone when I'm puking all the time.'

'What kind of kittens?'

'Two tabby, one black and white. One tortoiseshell. She's a mentalist, she's my favourite, likes going up the curtains. But we've got to sell them before they're allowed out or they'll all get squished on the road.'

'I've got a tabby but she'd hate a kitten, or I'd love one. Try a ginger biscuit, it might settle your stomach.'

She takes one, nibbles it and then puts it back on her saucer and clenches her hands.

'Can I just be knocked out for the birth, then?'

'I don't really know, I think you'd need to talk to a midwife about that. Or an obstetrician. Have you asked anyone so far?'

'*She* wouldn't tell me a thing except I didn't know what I was doing.'

I just sip my tea. I'm trying hard to do what Mum used to tell me: *don't try and feel their emotions for them*. I sometimes have the feeling that I can be a bit over the top. But I'm seething for her.

'That midwife's called Karen. She's a bitch. I went to see her and she said I had to make up my mind about whether I wanted to have the baby before I could find out anything about the birth.'

'Is that why you came tonight?'

'Yeah. I saw it on a leaflet in the midwife's office. I've given up fags and booze. I've started taking that vitamin, what's it called?'

'Folic acid?'

'Yeah. It makes me sick, but I take it. How am I supposed to decide for sure when I don't know what it's going to be like, though?'

Her voice has risen in agitation.

'Okay. You can definitely talk about all that with someone. How are you feeling about things besides the birth? Really?'

'It's just blood at this point, right, it's just a few weeks? A few months? So I could get rid of it.'

At ten weeks, a fetus has limb buds, eyes and ears and a beating heart. But I don't say this. Instead, I put an arm around her. Her face crumples and she starts to cry.

'I'm waiting for a scan. I dunno'.

I wait for a few seconds to see if there's anything more she wants to tell. Sometimes they just want to say it. But after a second she pushes me off and so I just sit there and wait for her sobs to subside.

Eventually, she sits up straight and breathes deeply, looking floppy and pale.

'Fucking awful,' she says. 'I'm never having sex again my whole life.'

'Look, I'm not a midwife, right? Just a volunteer? You need some proper support.'

'I don't want another midwife. She just looks at me like I don't know what I'm doing and okay maybe I don't, but isn't that her job? Isn't she supposed to be telling me? Giving me some fucking clues, at least?'

I rummage around in the red plastic box and find the leaflet about the teenage support team. I get a biro and write my own number on the back of the leaflet too. I also fish her out the ones on active birth, caesarean, delivering the placenta and pain relief.

'You really need to talk to someone. If you get stuck, ring me. But make an appointment. I can't help that much.'

She nods and smiles in a watery way and sips her tea. I relax a bit. I thought she might be angry at me for interfering. She's going to make decisions based on emotion, not anything else, so you have to make sure she respects herself for asking for help. In my opinion, Karen has got this bit of her care wrong so far.

'Thanks. So, I'm probably not doing this. I'd be a shit Mum.'

Her hand is resting on her belly under her messenger bag. I choose my words with care.

'Okay, so this pregnancy is a surprise. But that doesn't mean you'll be shit. If this is what you want, it could be the best thing ever.'

Out of the window, I see a car draw up. It's a yellow VW Beetle. An older woman with a shock of a white bob gets out, wearing a long black skirt, a grey sparkly cardigan, a crucifix and a lanyard. She's a big woman, she has a large bone structure and a large...well, everything really.

'Come and join the class if you like. It might help you decide. Labour is hard. But it doesn't have to be terrifying or what you can't handle. It's not like on TV.'

'How would you know?'

'My Mum used to be a home birth midwife. I've been to a few births.'

Her lip is curling again, ready to get defensive.

'We get Mums your age. Promise. If this lot are judgemental, that's their issue. Come and see?'

I think she's been spooked by the car; she's watching the woman move files and boxes around in her boot. I'm suddenly furious I can't start training this year. Who knows, I could have actually helped someone.

'No, I'm going to go, my bus is soon...'

'Okay. Well, I mean it. Call me if you get into difficulties. But you will make that appointment?'

She nods, looking tiny and ferocious. I follow her down the hall to the door.

'Good luck. Be really, really nice to yourself, okay?'

'Okay. See you,' she turns, as an afterthought, 'What's your name again?'

'Chloe.'

'Bye Chloe.''

'Bye.' I watch her disappear down the street, walking fast, pulling up her headphones and then her hood. Then I go out to see if the woman in the yellow Beetle needs a hand.

'Who was that then?' she asks, by way of greeting, now taking leaflets and blood bottles out of a black zip-up sports bag. I see from her ID that her first name is Enid and the word 'midwife', but it's too dark for me to see her full title. Her voice is lilting and Irish.

'She's called Sadie, she didn't come to the class. I think she just wanted someone to talk to, actually.'

She peers at me and frowns, 'Who are you? What's your name?'

'Chloe Cawthorne, I'm just a volunteer.'

'Cawthorne, is it? Aha, *just* a volunteer, I don't think so. Marie was your Mum, yes? And Daniel was her partner, your Dad. I know him from old.'

I stiffen, worried about how much she knows about him these days, but Enid doesn't seem to be implying anything.

'Does she have a midwife? This Sadie? Did you give her the details?'

'Yes. I gave her the teenage pregnancy clinic number.'

'Take this for me,' she hands me a box, 'Well, hopefully

she'll take your advice.'

We're walking in together now and my heart leaps into my mouth as the light catches her name badge. It has 'Senior lecturer, De Montfort University' written on it.

'So you're volunteering. Who is it, Karen on tonight taking the class? She's new here, isn't she?' I nod, 'How old are you? Are you wanting to be a midwife, like your Mum?'

I look up at her flat expression, wondering if she recognises my name from the application.

'I... I'm eighteen. And yes, though I haven't interviewed yet this year.'

'There's an interview on Thursday over on the main campus, it's for the cohort starting in March really, but you might just make the September start, could you do that at such short notice?'

I nod, holding my breath.

'Right. Good. It's in the Portland Building. What are your grades? Subjects? You got your A-level results last week, didn't you?'

'Um, yes. Chemistry, Biology, English. BAA.'

'Oh, very good, it'd be a shame not to have you then. And obviously, you've got experience.'

I let my breath out in a rush.

'Mm. You're not the one who wrote about *The Scientification Of Love* in your personal statement?'

'Um. Yeah.' I'm flushing.

'Yes, you're quite clued up, aren't you? You like Michel Odent? He has birthing rooms near Paris. He's a brilliant speaker, if you can ever get to a conference.'

'Yes. I know. I mean, I haven't seen him, but I'd love to go to a midwifery conference.'

'But why haven't you interviewed already? Am I missing

something?'

I think as fast as I've ever thought.

'I did have an interview invite. I thought I couldn't attend, we had some family stuff going on. But it should all be okay now. I was going to leave it until next year as I missed my interview –'

She interrupts me, looking bored like she doesn't need any more of anyone else's problems.

'Oh, don't be ridiculous, we need students like you now. Tell them I said it was fine. I won't be on the panel but I'll let them know you're coming.'

Holy hell. I can't cope with this.

We take a seat at the back of the hall and watch Karen talking the group through the possibility of needing stitches. She's talking about *'getting your bits and pieces back in the right place, sometimes you need senior members of the team in so we can make sure we've done it right'*. She's scaring them, I think, but I can't concentrate properly.

I'm sat here grinning and Karen keeps glancing at me, confused. I shut my eyes and I'm trembling with excitement. I decide I need to get some more sleep. That's what I'll do, before the interview. And choose my clothes. And re-read everything we have by Michel Odent and look through Mayes *Midwifery* and the *Changing Childbirth* report.

At the end of the class, I gather cups and stack chairs and I think Enid has left without saying goodbye. But then she makes me start as she taps me on the shoulder.

'Chloe. Here we go.'

She pushes a cloth drawstring bag into my hands.

'You can have this if you like. Found it at the back, I think it's been there a while. Do some reading on them before Thursday.'

'Oh, thanks.'

She looks at Karen, 'I'm off, Mrs Hodgson, if that's alright with you? The boxes are in the hall. I've got to catch up with a doctor over at the Royal...'

'That's fine, Chloe can help me clear up, can't you Chloe? She's a good girl!' she puts her hands on my shoulders. I can smell her perfume – heavy, like lilies. I wonder why she's acting like she's met me before, maybe she's trying to impress Enid. I step forward, out of her grip and shake Enid's hand, thanking her for the opportunity and trying not to sound like I'm sucking up.

As Enid leaves, Karen asks, 'I see, all this volunteering is because of your interview?'

'Mmm,' I say, non-committally.

'Well, good for you. Did I see that teenager, what's her name, hanging around?'

'Uh, yeah, Sadie? She was here. She didn't want to come into the main class though.'

Karen laughs unpleasantly and my heart sinks.

'She can be exceptionally rude and difficult. Was she alright with you? She didn't try to sell you a kitten, did she?'

'She was fine. Just scared. Maybe because she's closer to my age or something, perhaps she isn't as likely to give me a hard time...' I'm scrabbling to find the right thing to say and Karen looks irritated. Well, fine, actually, because I'm irritated with her. 'I gave her the teen pregnancy number, I hope that's okay?'

'Well, I think they're closing their doors soon, but she can try, I suppose. The funding's been cut. I'm not entirely sure she should be seeing midwives until she's decided on a termination or not, anyway.'

The last few couples are still chatting in the doorway and I don't want to be talking about this in a place where we can be overheard. I try and keep my expression neutral.

'Did she tell you what she's decided?'

'Not really. I think she just wanted to talk...'

'What did you get, then? What's in the bag?'

I open it. It's a pinard horn, like an elongated egg cup, eight inches long and made of a grained, pale cream wood. It's for listening to fetal hearts. Unlike the plastic, electronic sonicaids, these take a lot of skill to be able to hear a fetal heart at all, but the auscultation is real, rather than interpreted electronically. I saw Mum using one in America and I remember it the few times we had pregnant friends over and she had a listen in while they lay on the sofa.

I turn it in my hands and with a shiver, I see there are initials near the base. *M.C.* I know the wood-burning technique that's been used, it's something Dad gets paid commissions for. This was Mum's.

'Well it's not like you can be practising with that yet, but it's a nice thing to put in your room or something, I suppose,' says Karen, frowning.

'Mm.'

I put the pinard back, and into my rucksack, away from her. I'll look at it properly at home.

We go into the kitchen and I wash up the cups, while Karen dries them and puts them away and complains. Too much work, ungrateful women, arrogant students and her daughter becoming vegetarian are all on her list.

Then she says to me, 'How old are you again?'

'Eighteen.'

'Have you thought about doing something other than midwifery first? I'm not sure a lot of eighteen-year-olds know what they're getting into when it comes to midwifery, to be honest. I know you have a bit of experience here, but have you got anything hands on? Do you know what it's like day to day? Imagine going up the M1 resuscitating a baby with Mum looking on and knowing you aren't going to get a break once you reach the hospital...'

I feel like turning around and saying, *no, of course I don't know what that's like. And I don't think you know what it's like to be me either. Or a teenager who's pregnant.*

But I don't. There will be things I can learn from Karen, she's experienced. I concentrate on washing up. A film of soap has formed in the handle of one of the cups on the draining board and catches the light, making a rainbow on its transparent surface. Karen picks up the cup and the bubble breaks.

'I'd just consider things carefully if I were you. Some of these younger students –' She makes a small, unimpressed noise.

'Well, waiting a few more years before you start won't do you any harm at all, get your life sorted before you take on anything else.'

'I think Enid wants me to interview next week...?'

'Yes, well, Enid's encouraging. But life is complicated enough when you're eighteen, you're only just sorting out who you are, don't you think? Like my daughter.'

'My Mum was a midwife.'

I wasn't planning on saying this, but it pops out anyway. Karen stops drying.

'*Was?* Did she get struck off or something?'

'No... she died.'

'Oh, sweetheart, I'm sorry.' She doesn't sound that sorry at all. I don't want to talk about it but she asks, 'What was her name? And when did she...?'

'Marie Cawthorne. Coming up to three years ago now.'

'Oh Marie, yes, I knew her! She was a strong personality, wasn't she? And such a shock when she passed, no warning... You must have been very proud of her. Well, Chloe, I don't think there would be any disadvantage in terms of you taking another year and getting some proper experience. Travel, enjoy life. Get a bit of maturity under your belt...'

Her judgement for Sadie, along with my last few days with Dad, mounts up and suddenly I'm raging.

'Thanks for your advice. And your experience.'

She starts drying again. She's got the point, but there's nothing in her stance that's embarrassed. She's totally sure she's in the right.

4

Beginnings

It's the night before my interview and my bed has almost every piece of clothing I own piled up on it. I've tried dresses, trousers and ironed all my shirts and I'm just wasting time when I could be reading up. I wish I could just wear my healthcare assistant uniform. Nothing looks *right* apart from that.

Dad has been bumping around in the attic all afternoon. I'm surprised he's got the enthusiasm but glad he's got a focus. Now I think he's watching TV, they're running a summer evening film and I'm pretty sure it's *Die Hard*. I heard him join in with the 'yipee-yi-yea' line anyway.

In the end, I go for heels and a pencil skirt because at least they'll know I'm making an effort. I'm milk-bottle pale in a dark blue shirt and I look like a secretary. I want to call Jos to get her opinion, but she has a thing with Hamza tonight, it's some kind of wedding rehearsal. Weddings are like a sport for Hamza's family. Jos's collection of *shalwar kameezes* now outnumbers her jeans and t-shirts. Against my better judgement, I wobble down the stairs to ask for Dad's advice.

He's watching Bruce Willis stepping barefoot on glass with a gun duct-taped to his back that Alan Rickman doesn't know about yet.

'Dad?'

He turns with a bland TV expression and then smiles his best proud Dad smile.

'This is for your big day, then?' he says.

'Oh God, I'm not getting married or anything. I probably won't get it, please don't get excited. Is what I'm wearing alright?' I pull at the shirt to smooth it out.

'You look beautiful, yeah. You feeling ready for it?'

I just look at him.

'Oh, whatever, they'll never have seen anyone better. Come here,' I go over and he gives me a hug and I kiss his scratchy face and smell his recently cleaned teeth and hope against hope that he's better. He's taught one woodwork class, has done some night shifts and I've only smelled weed in the evening of late. Even his jumper looks clean. Ish.

'They'd be idiots not to let you in. Tell them that, from me.'

'Yeah, excellent strategy. *Give me a spot or I'll set Dad on you.* I've got something to ask you about actually, stay there,' I take my heels off and run back up to find the cloth bag that Enid gave me.

I come back down examining the pinard.

'Oh, yeah, I remember this. It's beech, I did it on the lathe and then varnished it,' he takes it from me and turns it over in his leathery hands. He has yellow nicotine stains on his fingers. 'Where d'you get it from? I thought we'd lost it.'

'Mum left it at the antenatal class I think.'

'Oh, right. Funny how things turn up. I bet she would have left it to you if she could.'

'She didn't have time.'

'No, we could have used a warning. D'you remember that Paris trip we were planning? Missed it by about six weeks, that was all.'

'We all did our best. We didn't know what was going to happen. Loads of people have high blood pressure, but not many die of a stroke, especially the first one. Like they said, there was probably a heart condition that they never picked up.'

'Yeah.'

He looks so sad that I can't stand it, so I say, 'Why d'you make it? She had one already, didn't she, that one in a dark coloured wood?'

'She bought that one, it was factory made. She wanted something more special to work with. Also,' he says, leaning back and looking self-important, 'she wanted a connection with it. Something handmade by me was far more likely to keep her clients safe. She believed in things like that.'

I snort. 'You two were right old hippies, weren't you?'

He smiles.

'And d'you know where the word hippy comes from?'

'Yes, I believe I have heard once or twice...'

'It's African Wolof language.'

'From a source I can't quite recall...'

'And it translates as "eyes wide open".'

'Does it, now,' I say.

'That was your Mum all over. She got at least sixty years into her forty. She'd be so excited about you interviewing.'

'Yes. I know.'

I've looked this up in the library and hippy doesn't mean that. It just started being used in the sixties, from 'hip' and someone added a 'y'. But I don't say this. It's a line he loves.

On the TV, Bruce shoots Alan, Bruce's wife falls into his arms and the credits roll. Dad turns the set off.

'Right. I'm going down the chippy, what d'you want?'

There's no part of me untouched by the effort he's making.

Thursday, 24th August 2000

There are ten of us sitting on plastic chairs in a little portacabin waiting to be called, our emotions spiralling around the room. We're coping by concentrating on each other, quietly chatting. I'm sitting next to Noelia, who is Spanish, about forty and stands out as she is dressed in a bright green kaftan and a pair of leather boots laced up to the knees.

'I have a grown up son,' she says, 'He's a man, now at university himself. Even though he lives with his Mamma at home. People think it's weird in this country, but it's better for money, he gets cooked for, I get to enjoy him...'

I tell her I live at home with my Dad so I don't think it's weird at all, though I don't fill in any details. Then I ask her about midwifery in Spain and she tells me it's medicalised.

'In England, you've noticed that when you assume birth will be normal, it's more often normal. This is magical, we need more of this thinking. It's not the fault of the men involved, but they screw everything up. Dr this and Dr that bossing women about. Midwives are handing the women the keys again.'

'Are you a feminist?' I ask, smiling.

'If you have a vagina and you want to be in charge of what happens to it, you are a feminist darling,' she replies. She says 'vagina' in a very long drawn-out kind of way, with a soft 'b' instead of a 'v'. It makes me giggle.

'I see. Are you nervous today?'

'Too old to be nervous,' she says, grinning. The sun is intense; it's shining through the open window. It lights up her brown curls and brown eyes, which are almost cinnamon-coloured.

'Well, you don't look old to me. I'm sure you'll be fearless.'

'At least, I will act it. This is the last interview session? I decided last minute that this was my year – what about you?'

I don't know what I'm going to say, but I'm glad I don't have to explain, as a midwife in a blue uniform opens the door and calls my name.

'Buena suerte!' Noelia grabs my hand as I go past and squeezes it. I decide I really like her.

The midwife walks me out of the portacabin across the campus. The sun is reflecting off the student union building, which is made of glass, red plastic boards and metal brackets. It looks ugly next to the old church. I remember marching across here with Christopher on that freezing cold night. It's a comforting thought: I was nervous then and it ended so well.

We walk through the Portland Building. It smells like floor polish and old books; there are plaster roses set around the ceilings and a marble floor. It's completely empty of students as it's summer and my heels echo. I'm having to work hard to keep up with the midwife when we get to the stairs; she's in sensible black work shoes. I should have worn trousers and flats. Midwives don't wear heels. I don't know what I was thinking, but it's too late now.

'Wait here, please.'

She leaves me outside a door. It's too warm, my head aches and I can feel sweat prickling under my arms. A chair scrapes and it makes me jump.

I close my eyes and I can almost see the words on the page. *'Vision 2000 is the Royal College of Midwives' campaign for normal birth document which outlines twelve key points...'*

'Chloe Cawthorne?' I snap my eyes open and manage to compress my anxiety into my stomach and follow the midwife into a carpeted classroom.

They've drawn the curtains to stop the sun coming in. Behind a long table sit three interviewers looking at a single chair.

A woman turns from another uniformed midwife she's been chatting to and then I have a moment of pure paralysis because it's Karen, *Karen*, in a frilly shirt, with a clipboard.

'Chloe! Come on in then, d'you want to take the hot seat?'

She looks and sounds thrilled. She nudges the midwife next to her, 'Look, the surprise on her face!' I swallow.

'I know Chloe from the Aylestone antenatal class. I'm one of the assessing mentors today, one dropped out so I volunteered. That's good isn't it, that we know each other? Don't be nervous!'

I try to smile back at her and feel myself grimacing.

I'm trembling, but I don't know if they can see it. I hope not, anyway. I'm not sure whether to shake hands but the midwife who walked me over has taken a seat and Karen says, 'Come on then, we'll get stuck in,' so I sit down.

I'm taken aback as she says, 'I'll start. I'm sure you won't be surprised by my first question. D'you feel old enough to be a midwife, Chloe? Do you know what the role entails?'

The midwife who walked me over coughs. She's frowning, looking through me, not at me. I wasn't able to take her in while we were walking, but she has grey hair and fine features and looks kind and tired.

She says, 'Do you need anything, Chloe? Usually we'd offer

you a glass of water before we start.' She nods at a jug on the table.

'No. I'm fine. Thanks. Um, the role of the midwife. It's not complicated. I mean – I don't mean that –'

It's just energy. That's what Mum would have said. It's just a load of energy in your stomach. Breathe with it.

I can see Karen out of the corner of my eye, seated on her cushioned chair, readjusting herself to be more comfortable. I look at her. And then I get angry and think, *fuck you. I'm not letting you do this to me.*

Something about my internal swearing seems to make Karen unsteady and her smile falters a bit.

I focus on the older midwife and answer.

'Well, I've been going to the antenatal class for a few years now... doing lots of listening to women. I'm an HCA at the Royal. I'm committed... and I care about every woman I come across.'

The midwife next to Karen has teardrop earrings, which look odd with her uniform. She's nodding.

'For instance, mentioning no names there's a teenager who came to the antenatal group –'

Karen interrupts.

'Oh, Sadie? Yes, she's a lost soul all right, she's got herself into a right mess. You talked for a long time, didn't you? I've got her in with the teenage pregnancy midwife for as long as *that* service lasts, anyway.'

I breathe. The other midwives on the panel are scribbling.

'Yeah. Okay. She needed someone to talk to. So that's what we did and I might not have ever been a pregnant teenager, but I've certainly felt lost and confused and unsure in my life, so I tried to remember what that felt like. And listen. And then the week before I was talking to a Mum who'd needed four rounds of IVF and of course I've not been there either. But...'

The midwife with the earrings is smiling at me, looking right into my eyes.

'I know a bit about nursing and midwifery's different. I want to be there across the whole thing, from when they find out they're pregnant, to the labour, to the postnatal care. Women are interesting. They should have options and truth and support... and if I could be part of that, it'd be amazing.'

'Right, well, I think we've got the point,' says Karen, 'Moving on.'

The older midwife massages her eyes with her fingers.

The rest of the interview goes so fast that I can't believe it when it's done. They didn't ask me nearly as much as I thought; they seemed more interested in what my feelings are, as opposed to facts. I didn't get to tell them about any of the reports I've read.

I shake their hands, then I'm let go.

After I walk out of the door I get confused and go the wrong way, up some more stairs to a corridor with a big window. I can see Noelia being walked over by the older midwife and I want to wave, but persuade myself I might not get a place if they see I've been wandering around the building on my own. Do student midwives need a good sense of direction?

I dart back down the stairs and walk home, possibly more anxious than I was during the interview.

When I get back home, a red light is flashing on the answer machine on the hall table. I try to remember if it was doing that this morning. Probably it was and I didn't notice because I was so nervous. I convince myself that it can't possibly be the university, it's far too soon and then when I listen to the message I panic. It's the admissions department, and they want me to ring them.

I know immediately that it is bad news. I shouldn't have been interviewed at all, it was a mistake of Enid's. I didn't put myself forward enough. They've found out about Dad.

I sit on the hall stool and dial three separate times, each time hanging up before it rings.

The fourth time, I tell myself to stop faffing about and let the call go through because this will be looking really bad to them if they can see the number. The nice woman in admissions tells me that the university wants to know if I can start in two weeks, and I accept and thank her with calm and professional composure and put the phone down.

I walk into the garden and sit on the mossy steps and watch the flowers in the breeze. After a while I put my hands over my face and when I take them away again, there's a beautiful sun-soaked sky, with clouds as flat and soft as a snowdrift.

I imagine Mum laughing at me, telling me off for worrying, *did you actually think it wouldn't happen, Chloe, my serious girl?* The moment is so fragile that I don't want to lose it and I sit there barely able to stand it.

Then I walk back into the house in which I was born and call everyone to let them know.

And so, I'm a student midwife.

First we're out at the Nursing and Midwifery campus, which is separate from the rest of the university and in a converted Victorian manor house. Everything feels slightly Hogwarts, with a stained-glass coat of arms in the front door and ivy climbing the walls.

Enid drifts in and out of our lectures. I often turn round and see her standing at the back like a big midwifery ghost with a crucifix. I'm not sure whether she's interested in how we're doing, or just wants it known that she could be anywhere and we'd better watch out. She never catches my eye.

Mostly it's induction stuff, manual handling and fire safety, which we do alongside the nursing and occupational therapy students. We all have terrible student IDs done – there's just one go at getting the picture, meaning we're all squinting and startled.

But we are shown a video of a birth one morning, an oxytocic dream of a birth with a midwife with a plastic apron over her jeans and t-shirt and the woman in her living room. The woman is yelling on her hands and knees and when the baby is born his cries chime in with hers, she rocks back on her feet and receives him through her legs. She laughs in disbelief and looks up at whoever's holding the camera, like *yeah, how amazing am I!*

As she's stroking his velvet head I'm captivated, but when the lights come back on a girl with straight black hair has packed her things into her bag and walks out there and then. We hear her say to the lecturer, 'I wasn't sure, but now I am. This is so not for me.'

For the September to December modules we're in uni full time and I'm in love with the course. On Tuesdays and Thursdays, Dad's up before I go. He's banging around in his shed a lot, supposedly making demos for his woodwork class, so I make him eat toast with me before he goes out.

Then I walk to college and meet the small group of girls that I've fallen in with, the freaks and geeks that are as enthusiastic about birth as me.

We differ. Ada is German and blonde and pragmatic. Mehreen is reliable and sweet. She's into fashion and I've never seen her in the same outfit twice.

Noelia also got in. She's my favourite new friend. Her

clothes are handmade, eclectic and brightly coloured, and she has 'extravagances' like a hot drink and a pastry every morning from the café. Ada, Mehreen and I join her in this to begin with, but we all agree that it starts to add up money-wise and I think I can see my tummy start to bulge after a few weeks. I don't know how Noelia gets away with it.

This is what Noelia is like: when we have to present back to the class about handwashing theory, she whoops and claps when the first group have finished. She stops clapping when she realises she's all on her own, appalled at our lack of enthusiasm. But the lecturer restarts the applause and the class follow, laughing a bit. Noelia whispers to me, 'You English, you're weird, so embarrassed about everything...'

The only midwifery-specific lectures we have at this point are on anatomy and physiology and I cover my room with drawings, having gone to the uni bookshop to buy an art pencil set with as many colours as I can find. The way embryos develop is complex, subtle, origami-like. They're not pretty, but they don't have to be at this stage, I suppose. They're designed to be deep inside.

We get to pick our first essay topic and I choose 'The midwife and informed choice' and write about Down's Syndrome. It's a challenge because we can only do a thousand words with just five references, but I can't get frustrated. I'm thrilled all the time. Christopher and Dad and Jos have noticed and tease me about smiling. If I'm staying round Christopher's, I'm not allowed to enthuse about anything midwifery-related before he's finished his first cup of coffee in the morning.

On uniform day there's a hum in the air as we mill around waiting for free bathroom stalls. It feels like the first dress rehearsal of a school play as we open plastic packets with less enthusiasm than we were hoping for. Even in the extra small size, they don't skimp on material; I have no idea why some people find this kind of outfit sexy. They're pretty appalling, just a light blue tunic with no real shape, two slanted pockets and a zip up the middle.

Everyone is taking turns to look at themselves in the full-length mirror in the hall. A quiet black female lecturer in a rose cardigan is watching us. When it's my turn I go into the cubicle, put on a tunic and the navy trousers and fix my hair with grips. I also take off my necklace and rings, which you can't have on the ward because of infection control. I want to see the full effect.

When I come and look into the mirror I see the tunic is far too big. I could camp out in it. Noelia, Ada and Mehreen giggle at me.

'It's alright for you guys. You have boobs to fill them out,' I say, turning to catch the light.

'They're okay,' says Ada, 'They look... professional.'

'You all need darts put in,' says Noelia. 'Take them off. Come round Friday, I'll give them shape, no problem. You'll all look gorgeous.'

'You already look gorgeous,' says Mehreen.

'Thanks,' I say softly, still looking at myself, 'I'll take them to my Nanna's, she'll want to do them. But thanks for the offer.'

Nanna was a machinist for a while and then did some sewing freelance. She's good at that kind of thing.

'We've got months before we need them. Are you all not bored of uni? Why can't we do more on the wards earlier? I want to be out there delivering babies, not just discussing it for hours...' Ada starts moaning.

I remember Mum ranting at some midwifery convention thing I was taken along to as a kid. She said midwives shouldn't wear uniforms and that they were a combination of a nun's habit and something military, and we like to lord it over women in them. Still though, I'm excited. Unlike the candy-striped dress that picked me out as a healthcare assistant, the plain light blue will be the first colour I ever wear to catch a baby in. I turn in the light and, despite the fit being awful, I get a glimpse of myself as the women might see me. I look capable, a new version of myself. Everything is beginning.

Saturday, 9th December 2000

The tiny brick house is on the edge of the village, the chimney always trickling out smoke in a thin, unfurling column. In the summer the fields are full of corn, but it's winter so I think it's turnips now. That's what the fields smell like, anyway.

I've come to see Nanna with Jos, something we often do together now I've inherited Mum's Ford and can drive over to Desford. It's Saturday morning, before my evening healthcare assistant shift. Sunday would be a much easier time to visit, but Nanna always goes to church, a three-mile walk each way.

Nanna's got me standing on a stool and is putting pins into one of the uniforms, which still looks to me like a blue lampshade with pockets, but I have high hopes that when she's finished you may actually be able to see I've got a waist.

Through the net curtain the long garden is full of bamboo stakes left over from the summer. Everything is dying back. Nanna looks like she could snap in two, but this is just her disguise; she grows food and makes jam and pickle for herself and half of Desford and runs all the societies from her kitchen table with brisk efficiency.

Her face is flushed and her glasses reflect the coals glowing through the stove window. Her fuel allowance, being a miner's widow, means her house is like the centre of the earth. I remember Ali and me misbehaving round here when we were little because we got overheated and it made us grumpy.

'When I finished school you were expected to get a trade and that was that. Hatched, matched and dispatched they called it. It's clever, getting paid for an education and being a midwife at the same time.'

'Don't go telling anyone I'm a midwife yet! I've got to get through three years before I can call myself that.'

'Oh yes, don't worry, I won't say. And what about you Jocelyn, what are you doing at university?'

'Graphic design, Nora,' Jos is flopped in one of the armchairs sipping tea from a gold-rimmed china teacup patterned with hydrangeas. She took her headscarf off in the car, thank God. I don't think I could do the Islam conversation with Nanna.

'Goodness. That does sound exciting.'

Nanna darts off into the dining room and comes back with a tape measure. She stands back to admire me.

'Just like your Mum. I never did know where she got her cleverness from...'

'I think you had a lot to do with it, didn't you, Nanna?'

'Hmm? Oh, no. Your Mum marched to the beat of her own drum, right from when she were little.'

Yeah, I think and *you handed her the sticks*, but I know there's no point saying it, she'll never take compliments, though she gives them all the time.

'And how's your sister?' There's a slight edge to Nanna's voice. I know this means that she hasn't seen Ali in months.

'She's working hard, teaching lots of classes. I'll tell her to pop round. She's just busy right now,' Nanna nods and leans in to measure around my bust. Up close she smells of talcum powder and the cold earth she's been digging in the garden.

'That's good, isn't it? When do you need these dresses?'

'In January. That's my first placement.' My stomach lurches and excitement rises in my chest.

'Oo, how wonderful! Where's that then?'

'Labour ward. Loads of girls have their first placement in the community, which slides you in a bit more gently, but I suppose it's a good thing. It's all experience. I'll get to catch babies.'

Time is disappearing at the moment, moving me from uni to Christopher's house to healthcare assistant work and back again, impossible to hold on to. At night I close my eyes and wake up two seconds later with the sun streaming through the windows. I know Christmas will disappear into the air like the smoke from Nanna's chimney.

'You'll love it, just like your Mum. You're both made for it. She used to cycle back here on a Friday night when she was doing her midwifery and just talk at me for hours, telling me about this baby and that baby... and your Dad's lucky to have you. How is he?'

She turns away and rummages in a drawer, her back hunched. Jos sets her teacup down with care, giving me a look.

'Yeah, he's doing much better, Nanna.' It's not really a lie. He does seem a bit more with it at the moment.

I'm furious with him for chasing Nanna away though. It's awful, because she's bereaved too, and Dad and she both need the family they have left. She used to come round for a brew when she did her Leicester shopping, but she knows there's something deeply wrong that she can't help with going on in the house these days, so she keeps her distance. At least she has her church friends. This is especially important at Christmas. Last Christmas for us was a disaster. Dad and Ali got high and

Ali whited out and threw up everywhere.

'Oh, before I forget, I've got a little wreath of Christmas roses in for your Mum. Fake ones, but they'll do until the poinsettia's ready. Can you put them out for me?'

Mum's buried in the Desford graveyard.

'Thanks, that'll look lovely. We'll drive over on our way back.'

'Is your Dad working?'

'Sometimes.'

'He's had his troubles. All that sleeping during the day did him no good at all, though.'

She slides one more pin into the bottom of the tunic and then waves at me to get down.

'How's your Mum, Jocelyn? And your young man?' Jos shifts in her chair and I unzip myself carefully so I don't get pricked by the pins. I change back into my jeans and jumper. I'm grateful for this time, the warmth, the sound and shape of the conversation and the fire popping and crackling.

Jos is telling Nanna a censored version of the Hamza dilemma and Nanna is nodding sympathetically. I haven't told Nanna about Christopher. I'm not sure what she'd think about his age. It's getting more uncomfortable though. I'll have to tell her at some point. It's exhausting remembering to stay on safe ground.

'It's Hamza I'm most worried for, he's got to make his Mum happy and I respect him for that of course, but it's his life. Y'know, marriage lasts for a whole lifetime...'

'I didn't realise it was so serious, dear. Aren't you both a bit young to be thinking about marriage?'

'How old were you when you got married?'

'Oh, I see, true. Er. But it was a different time, love...'

'I'm desperate, to be honest Nora, I don't know what to do.'

'Well dear, if it's meant to be, it'll work out. That's what we always said.' She disappears into the kitchen. Jos sits back in her chair, looking devastated.

I put one hand on hers and whisper 'She doesn't mean it, she just doesn't know what to say.'

Nanna comes back in with three bowls with the same hydrangea pattern as her tea cups and one small blue jug she uses for cream and I know we're about to be fed a lot of calories. She puts on a thick pair of oven mitts with cats on and opens the hatch at the top of the stove and I make a little sound. I know the smell well, there's a rice pudding in there.

She heads back into the kitchen to get the jam.

'That's amazing Nanna, pudding for breakfast.'

'Well, I've eaten my breakfast hours ago, this is lunch for me. D'you not want some now?'

We'd never refuse, she'd be so offended. But then again, we don't want to. Even Jos cheers up a bit.

'Maybe take some back for your Dad, too. He always looks so thin...'

Nanna sets the dish on the cork mat and serves us huge portions, the rice oozing thick hot milk. It's such a reassuring food, I've loved it since before I can remember and back when I was a kid she used to buy pink sugar to have on it, probably full of horrible colourings that made Ali and me hyper. There's a silence as we all start eating.

Then we start giggling because the quiet goes on and Jos and I are shovelling far more jam and syrup and sugar into our bowls than is strictly ladylike.

This is a lot easier than having conversations about boys and badly behaved family. I look out into Nanna's garden and can see the spire of the church, the stones of which are standing invisible below the tree line. I wonder if I'll ever have my life as sorted as Nanna. I'll try.

5

Initiation

It's my first ever shift on labour ward and I am a ball of excitement and stress. As I follow the plastic signs through the Leicester General Hospital, my flat, sensible shoes squeak on the lino.

I know from inspecting myself in the mirror that, thanks to the magic of Nanna, for the first time in my NHS career I look quite pretty. I know that looking professional is way more important than attractiveness, that the women won't care at all, but still, I'm grateful for any extra confidence that I can scrape together and my pale blue uniform skims over my hips, showing I'm not just a little girl.

I'm hit by a wave of hospital cleanliness. The smell of antiseptic and lemon air freshener triggers a memory. The last time I was in this hospital was more than five years ago. I was picking Mum up from work with Dad. I remember Mum being furious about something and this makes me worry a bit. I remind myself to take it slowly, shift by shift. There might be stuff that I find hard to take.

I buzz at the labour ward door and it takes them a few

minutes to answer. It's a healthcare assistant, one I don't recognise; she probably just works here rather than at the Royal as well. It's reassuring to see her familiar uniform, but she doesn't know this. I must look as young and green as they come.

She shows me the changing-room and tells me the keycode. 'Write it down and keep it safe, duck,' she advises me and when I've put my coat and sandwich away, she drops me off at the handover desk.

I look at the gridded whiteboard. I don't know much, but it looks more like a mission to Mars than a lot of women having babies. EDD, ECC, NVD. Synto. That must be syntocinon, the artificial version of the labour hormone oxytocin. I've read about it. There seems to be a lot of that going on this evening.

I check my fob watch, my new silver one with the glow in the dark face that Jos got me for Christmas. Fifteen minutes to wait. I should have arrived later. I've given myself time to fret. The excitement is turning to adrenaline, making my stomach tighten around the cereal I ate for dinner; I haven't done twelve-hour night shifts before and this, as much as anything else, is worrying me.

I look around to distract myself. The corridors are lined with drip stands and equipment trolleys and there isn't any natural light. The porthole windows on the birth room doors remind me a little of something military, the under-decks of a boat, or inside a submarine. The antiseptic smell is stronger here, mingled with the richness of instant coffee from the kitchen. As a woman and a man go past, both in blue scrubs, I notice their voices and footsteps echo.

I catch something about *'that one in four, best to keep her on side'* and then they both disappear into a room off the corridor and the door slams behind them. Something about their unsure expressions and sheer exhaustion makes me suspect that they're new too. Junior doctors, probably.

A woman approaches the board and looks it over. I glance over at her; she's also in scrubs, with glossy black hair done up in an elegant twist, topped with a silver butterfly clip. She's not pretty exactly, more handsome, with high, square cheekbones.

'Busy...' she says. 'We're in for a chaotic night I think.' She sighs, slouching to one side, running her thumbnail down a folded piece of paper in her hands, over and over.

'Mmm,' I say, without commitment. Her accent is from a well-to-do family, like Hamza's.

'How are the twins getting on?' she asks.

'Sorry, I don't know,' I say. She looks over, puzzled, clearly wondering why I'm not aware of such an important fact, and then she starts and smiles.

'Hang on, I know you! Who was that midwife... Marie Cawthorne? You're one of her daughters. You look like her. I know you from coming to her...'

She seems a little awkward and I realise she's talking about Mum's funeral. Sometimes people need permission to talk about that kind of thing, so they know I can cope. I'm resigned; I was planning not to mention who I was to anyone, but I guess it was silly to think I'd get away with it.

'Yeah, sorry, I'm sure I'd recognise you too, but we had so many people there...'

'Yes, so many it was standing room only, wasn't it? She was a lovely midwife, Marie. Loved and missed. She was such a hard worker...' she holds her hand out and I shake it.

'I'm Dr Roshni, obstetric registrar. I was a locum when your Mum was here.'

'Chloe. Student midwife. This is my first year. First shift on labour ward, actually.'

I don't want there to be any misunderstandings about this. I also want to get the attention off me so I ask, 'Did you work somewhere else as well then? Locum means you were just here off and on, doesn't it?'

'Oh, no. I just took it slowly while my boys were small. I've been in Leicester for a long, long time.'

She looks me up and down and puts a hand just under the v-neck of her scrubs, touching her chest. 'Amazing. It makes me quite emotional to think about it. She'd be so proud of you.'

I smile awkwardly and hope she doesn't tell anyone else, as nice as this is. I'd rather be anonymous. I'm grateful as midwives in navy blue uniform dresses start to appear around us, yawning, drinking instant coffee and discussing last night's shift.

One midwife in navy is standing in front of the board, peering at it and muttering to herself. I take her to be the senior on.

'Who's mentoring you tonight?' Dr Roshni asks.

'I'm not sure.' The mentor I was going to have is on long-term sick leave, so although we're supposed to know who we're assigned before starting a placement, this hasn't happened.

Dr Roshni looks around as if she's going to recommend someone, but the senior midwife leans over the desk and taps her on the shoulder, 'Roshni. They were after you in room three, did you get there?'

'Yes, yes, evening Beth. I'm on my way.'

Then she beams at me and says, 'See – busy! A great first shift for you. Good luck!'

'Thanks.'

Beth announces, 'Right, we'll start handover,' and the

conversation dies away, all eyes on the board.

'Amelia Neate, Room One. Gravida two, para one, labile blood pressure, proteinuria. Started on induction this morning...'

I'm listening but I hardly understand a thing. I was hoping some of my knowledge would transfer from HCA work, but it seems I'll be starting from scratch. I keep my expression polite and attentive.

'We're waiting an hour for descent. Farida if you'd like to take her and get her pushing after that...'

The women are divided up and handed to the midwives and some start to drift into rooms.

'And we'll leave the final induction until tomorrow. She won't be happy about it, but it can't be helped.'

The senior midwife rounds on me and I see her eyes are wide. She has the look of a woman who know she'll be going hell for leather all night. I smile but she doesn't return it, just asks what stage of training I'm at, so I explain myself as fast as I can.

'And no mentor so far?'

'No, I was supposed to have Dina, I think.'

'She's off. Right – Jo?'

Another midwife ambles over. She's a head taller than Beth with a short, grey boyish haircut and is old, elderly even, but her eyes are sharp and alert. She smiles at me. For some reason, she reminds me of Julie Andrews and I relax a bit.

'Can you take –' Beth peers at my name badge, 'Chloe, please. Room four is the tricky customer who's very intent on a normal birth and since that's supposed to be what we're giving them in their first year training...'

Beth trails off and Jo puts a cool hand on my shoulder. She radiates epic calm as she says, 'First shift on labour ward and they've given you a night! Well, we'll be gentle with you, then, yes?' She steers me towards the corridor.

'Um, thanks. That'd be nice.'

'Have you done any other placements? You're what, four months into your training now? But no labour ward experience?'

'Uh. No...' I don't want to come across as a total rookie. 'But I was a healthcare assistant at the Royal, Ward 15 mostly...'

Beth overhears and turns around again, fast, breaking off her conversation with a tiny midwife who has been checking a bag of fluid with her.

'Oh, Chloe, d'you know how to clean rooms?'

'Sure,' I say, 'And do I obs. And bed baths. And I make tea and coffee, too.'

This makes her laugh and I grin back.

'Could I ask you to change room six for me, before the night gets started properly? Cheeky, but all our healthcare assistants are already off getting on with things.'

'No problem. Where's the cleaning trolley and the laundry?'

'Everything's in the linen cupboard and there's the sluice with the trolley right next to it. Ask Jo if you need anything. Thanks.'

The phone starts to rings and Beth picks it up and answers and gestures to me to get going. So I do.

The room is pretty horrible, with blood that I need to scrub off that's dripped down in between the sections of the bed. It takes me the best part of ten minutes to work out how to get the footrests at the bottom of the bed to fold away. They don't tend to have these on the elderly ward, so I don't know what I'm doing.

I wipe all the bits of the sectioned mattress and then mop the floor, clear away all the litter (mainly Monster Munch packets) and put new bin bags in each of the different bins, for dirty laundry and general rubbish and clinical waste, and hope it's all the same colour code system as at the Royal.

I have to ask where the disposal room is and by the time I've put the cleaning trolley away everything is dry and I can make the bed. I do it like we would on Ward 15, making sure the draw sheet, the smaller bit of material under the patient that can be removed, is over the gap where the bits of the mattress meet. I then tuck in the sheets and a blanket and plump the pillows.

I'm glad there's a big window in here. It makes it much more welcoming. I leave it open to get some air through, despite the drizzle. It's dark as the middle of the night already, but the birds are still singing.

There's a big apparatus in the corner with heater bars at the top and a tiny bag and mask for resuscitating babies. A trolley with a few sterile packs, bowl sets, syringes and needles stands in the corner. I wonder what happened in here. Not much seems to have been touched apart from the bed.

It looks tidy, but I bet I've done something they'd class as wrong, or at least not what would be expected. Every ward has different rules. Over on Ward 15 we use plastic draw sheets for obvious reasons, and the matron would have her shotgun out if she found us using cotton ones. She'd think it was a waste.

I smile. I know some students would moan that they were being used, that they shouldn't be doing the cleaning, that it's a waste of time that could be spent learning, especially on their first shift. But I feel useful, not something I was expecting tonight, and I'm grateful.

I knock gently on the door to Room Four and Jo lets me in.

It's the same setup as the room I've just cleaned but softened, the air thick with moisture, dark and with little star-shaped flickers of multicoloured light chasing each other over the walls. I look around and see a projector on one of the trolleys.

There's a solid white birth pool, which looks like it's been put into the room as an afterthought, with not enough space between it and the back cupboards. Another source of light is from soft, yellow-tinged lamps under the water, making the pool glow in a fairytale kind of way.

The woman in the pool has curly red hair and a Pink Floyd t-shirt, a black one with a prism splitting light into a rainbow. She's strong and well-muscled, though she's carrying quite a bit of weight, with a rounded, pink-tinged face. A yellow plastic duck is floating in the water beside her.

'Hello,' I whisper.

She's making a low moaning sound with her mouth open and her eyes closed. The noise sounds like she's concentrating rather than in pain.

'Hi,' says Jo, in a louder voice, sat at the table with the notes. 'This is Brenna. And Bob.'

Bob waves, I hadn't taken him in sat in the corner. He's wearing a baseball cap on backwards.

'Um, that room will need checking I think Jo, I don't know about restocking or anything yet...'

'I'm sure Beth will have thought of that,' she replies.

She waves me over to a stool and asks, 'Have you ever done a waterbirth before?'

'Not really,' I say, remembering a few pool births. Mum was acting illegally in Alabama and I was five, so it's a bit too complicated to talk about.

'Lots of the older midwives won't do them,' says Jo, sniffing. 'They won't update. You ones as you come through training will change all that. The main thing is to keep the temperature steady, you can be in charge. We'll check every fifteen minutes and write it down.'

She points at the pool and I see the duck has a little screen set on its back with a thermometer read-out.

'When Brenna's pushing we'll need to get the temp up to over thirty-five, because if it's cold the baby can gasp. Supposedly, they can mistake cold water on their face as air. We've talked about all that, though, haven't we Brenna? You can try and do a listen-in. That is, if Brenna doesn't mind, Chloe,' she adds.

'I don't mind,' says Brenna, leaning back on the side of the pool and opening her eyes. From her accent she's American. I hadn't realised.

I introduce myself and she gives me the thumbs up and then peels off her wet shirt and drops it over the side of the pool where it lands with a plop. Bob gets up and puts it in a carrier bag and mops up the water with a towel. They seem unsurprised to see me so Jo must have told them a student was coming.

Brenna is now naked, reclining on the pool wall, her breasts floating and her taut bump under the water white and freckled. I wonder whether she's naturally red-headed. She has that colouring, though the rest of her body hair is brown.

She starts contracting again, her crooning beginning low and rising in pitch. It's weird. This shift is new in many ways, but I'm overcome by the sound of her and the musky smells of sweat, wet hair and something else unidentifiable. Maybe high levels of hormones. I have a wave of nostalgia hit my stomach, the same hot excitement that I remember from being five and clinging on to Mum's leg while she was doing something with a woman. That sort of New Year party feel of being at a labour, up late and hanging out with lots of excited family.

Jo nods her head towards the door.

'I don't want to disturb you, Brenna. Chloe and I will just pop out for a sec so I can tell her what's happening.'

We go out into the light and I blink, coming back to reality. Jo smiles at me and flicks to the start of the notes.

'Okay, so the general idea with this lady is that she's going to do exactly what she wants. She declined induction... do you know what gestational diabetes is?'

'I've heard of it.'

'It's diabetes that occurs in pregnancy. Brenna's blood sugars are good, she's well controlled and it's not severe, but this is a big baby on board and she's just on the cusp of overweight, so the guidelines say we should have her on the monitor...'

'Okay...'

'Let's go back to the beginning. See this page, it's a summary sheet. Her first two were born at home, no diabetes then...' Jo runs her finger down the page, showing me where to find the basics and the words *advised against home birth* and *patient informed trust cannot support her* jump out at me.

'There's a risk of shoulder dystocia and she knows that too. Do you know what that is?'

'The baby's shoulders get stuck during the birth, with just the head out?'

'Yes. Well done. That's one of the scariest situations to find yourself in, in the whole of obstetrics. Now, we should be listening to this baby all the time, have her on the monitor, but Brenna doesn't want that because she wanted to be in the pool. With cardiotocograph monitoring she'd have to lie on the bed so we could put the straps on, and this is what the guidelines say to do because gestational diabetes means more risk of complications. But we're doing intermittent auscultations with the hand-held sonicaid. It's her choice, but the doctors think it's more dangerous. Does that make sense?'

'I think so,' I say. I'm not certain how Jo feels about this. She's cool and matter-of-fact.

'I'll call another midwife in when this baby's about to be born and if anything *does* happen, just stand to one side and let us get on with it, okay? Maybe look after Bob.'

'Okay,' I think my expression may be a bit shocked, but Jo's not looking at me, she's more interested in the scan and a graph.

'It's a complicated one and the doctors aren't happy....'

I don't think I've taken everything in, it's confusing. Surely the doctors should be okay if Brenna's signed everything? Isn't it her choice? And isn't normal birth less work for them anyway, especially if they're needed elsewhere on the ward?

'She'll have this pool birth. She's only four centimeters at the moment but labouring well, good for her! This'll be one for you to write a reflection on. Any questions?'

I shake my head and she grins at me. I follow her back into the quiet of the birth room.

By 1am, a storm has broken outside, with wind and rain whipping at the windows. Bob is sleeping in his chair with his feet on the table, his baseball cap the right way on and pulled down over his eyes. He's snoring quietly, which adds to the ambience. They've brought mix CDs with them and I'm enjoying the music. It's not anything I recognise, but is soft and beat driven.

Brenna has not long been examined by Jo. She's seven

centimetres and thrilled about it. Jo asks me if I know what well-effaced means, and I answer with such enthusiasm that they all laugh, but I'm excited because this baby is going to be born on my shift, I just know it. Well-effaced means a thin cervix, the baby's head pressing on it, telling the body that the cervix needs to disappear, to be pulled up by the bottom of the uterus, so the baby can descend.

Jo hovers as I wash my hands, put on latex gloves and draw up the saline and connect the syringe to the opaque plastic tubing that disappears into Brenna's arm. I've never flushed a drip before though I've seen it done many times. It's to keep the line open and working.

Brenna has her eyes closed as I push the fluid through under the dressing and mutters 'Horrible thing...'.

'Yeah, I know. Does it hurt? How are you doing?'

'I'm coping. I hate needles though. I'd take more contractions over that.'

'You're so amazing.'

She bares her teeth at me and grunts. Bob jumps, with a sound that I can imagine a walrus making, and sits up, blinking and stretching.

Brenna says, 'Honey, that's not a very attractive noise.'

'Sorry, babe.'

Jo catches my eye and smiles and then the music changes and Bob says, 'Oh yeah, this is a tune...' and starts twitching his leg and doing a drumbeat in mid-air.

It is a gorgeous song, the low velvet vocal underset with guitars and mixing with the sound of heavy rain outside our window. The lyrics are about driving and city lights.

I check the temperature of the pool water and it's a little cool so I let some out and add some warm. Then I wash and dry my hands and rub hand cream into them. They get sore when I do a row of shifts and tonight they're getting wet a lot and I've vowed to keep them healthy, through my whole career, hopefully. I come and sit next to Bob who's singing now. He knows all the lyrics, but hitting the notes seems optional.

'Who's the artist?' I ask.

'Oh, you don't know her?' he says, breaking off. 'This one's from old. It's Tracey Chapman.'

'Tracey? She's a she?'

'Yeah, it sounds like a guy, doesn't it? I thought that the first time I heard her. She's more well known in America. Brenna's from Chicago.'

'Oh cool. D'you ever get back there?'

'Yeah, her family are out there. We've been with our eldest, our little girl, but not our son. We'll have to go back when this little one's ready to fly. Our son likes this song, he dances to it.'

Bob puts his arms in the air and jiggles up and down to imitate.

'Cute.'

'Yeah. If only he was like that all the time... I don't suppose you'd like a toddler? Free to a good home?'

'Um. I think you're about to add another one to the family?'

'Yes, good point. We could have a one in, one out policy, though.'

Brenna's contraction finishes and she rests her arms and forehead on the side of the pool.

'When I was five, my family lived in Alabama for a year,' I venture.

Jo raises her eyebrows but keeps writing in the notes. Bob responds, 'Oh yeah? You remember much?'

'Not really. Huge cornfields. Blue skies and nice people.'

'I've never been down that far South, but that sounds about right. They have some troubles but it's a great place.'

'Troubles?'

'Oh, all kinds of things. Not to say we don't have racism in the UK, we absolutely do, but it's much more subtle.'

'The whole race dynamic was interesting. I remember Mum talking about that while I was growing up, I think she was really struck by it.'

Unbidden, a memory rises of Mum at a big midwifery convention. I don't remember exactly what it was for, but black feminist rights were involved. I remember being just about the only white kid there apart from Ali.

'Uhuh.'

'And the pancakes.'

'Oh yeah, the food is just amazing. I went there first of all back in the late eighties and when you grow up in Manchester on meat and two veg...'

Jo breaks in, 'Right, Chloe, do you want to do the next listen-in? I think you've done enough of putting your hands over mine. D'you think you can find it on your own?'

'Um,' I feel bad about being inept at this, but Brenna is already leaning back and getting herself lined up for me. I take the sonicaid off the table, slowly, and get myself positioned kneeling next to the pool.

I immerse the plastic handle into the water and turn the unit on. It makes a horrible screeching noise and I apologise and turn it off again until I've got it all in the right place. I lean over Brenna's bump, coloured stars travelling across me and the water and the wall and I flick the switch again, holding my breath. A crackling rhythm fills the room.

'Count for a minute,' says Jo.

With the lights and the music, this could be a moment for sentimentality, but I shake it off and look at my fob watch.

I count. When the minute is up I say, 'One three six?'

because there have been one hundred and thirty-six beats.

'Yep, no probs.' The heartrate sounds like a distant train rushing over tracks and it starts to speed up.

Jo grins at me. 'That's good and healthy, you found an acceleration. This baby's not bothered about labour, Brenna. And you found it fine, Chloe, well done. You'd usually palpate beforehand to find out where to listen. This baby's coming down, you're getting it quite low aren't you?' I'm holding the probe to Brenna's left, just before the line of her pubic hair starts.

'Can you get a pulse as well?'

Without letting go of the sonicaid, I feel for Brenna's hand, putting two fingers on her wrist. The rhythm is much slower than the baby's heart rate, maybe half as fast.

I count for a minute and tell Jo it's about ninety and then ask if I can let Brenna go as she's wiggling her hips and starting to moan again. I dry the sonicaid and put it away.

'This labour's textbook so far. What's the pool temperature?' Jo asks.

As I'm about to tell her, Brenna dips her head, grits her teeth and makes a low noise from her gut.

I look at Jo. 'Is that –?'

She nods, silently, smiling back at me, then says to Bob, 'She's doing great. You should be really proud of her.'

'Always am. She's a tough cookie.' He's digging through their bag for something. I watch him as he gets out a plain cream baby grow and a matching hat, which he lines up on the resuscitaire, to warm up under the lights. He knows exactly what he's doing.

Something about the experienced competence of his movements floors me in a way I'm not expecting. As he checks everything is back in Brenna's bag, does the zip up and slides it away under the bed so no one will trip, I'm nearly in tears and I don't know why.

'How's Room Four, then?' says Beth, sat at the staff base and printing blood forms off the computer as she listens to Jo's update.

I know I'm smiling like a lunatic, my feet barely meeting the floor. I'm having major déjà vu. I have a particular memory from a birth in Alabama where I was woken in the night, picked up under the arms and plonked down in front of the pool to see the baby born. I've always wondered why Mum thought this was something I needed to see, and whether I'd ever do it with my own child. I never thought to ask her before she died. Since then it's been a bittersweet thought, a touchstone for pride, regret, sadness and passion that I've come back to thousands of times. Tonight it's clearer than it's ever been.

Dr Roshni appears at the end of the corridor, some notes in one hand and a cardboard cup of tea and a KitKat in the other. I notice she's changed her shoes for black wellies. She must be coming out of theatre.

'How's it going?' she asks me.

'Yeah, very good. The woman in there is amazing.'

'Oh yes? This is the one that refused monitoring isn't it?' She takes a sip of her tea, flicks to the correct page in her notes and starts writing at speed.

'She declined being on the CTG, yes,' says Jo, reasonably. 'Chloe's doing listen-ins, aren't you Chloe? All the makings of a great midwife already.'

I beam at her.

Dr Roshni frowns. Some of her hair has fallen from her clip and she brushes it out of the way and asks, 'Fetal heart okay?'

'Beautiful, as far as intermittent auscultation goes.'

'Does she know the implications of what she's choosing, though?' says Beth, and my euphoria fades as I tune into the worried lines around her eyes.

Dr Roshni adds, 'I can come and speak to her, if you like. She knows me from the clinic and knows what my opinion is. Healthy Mum, healthy baby is what everyone wants.'

'I don't think a chat's necessary, but thank you. Brenna knows everything she needs to. She's signed the informed consent.' There is the barest edge to Jo's voice. 'She says she'll get out of the pool and go on the monitor if there are any problems, but at the moment everything looks and sounds great.'

Dr Roshni stops writing and glances first at Jo, then at me. I gulp at the brightness of her look, feeling a bit like a mouse about to be swooped down on by an eagle.

'If the patient has consented to monitoring if there is a problem, then I would find a problem.'

She says this with such care that I feel the weight of each syllable and my mouth falls open.

Jo nods, thoughtfully.

'I don't think we need your input yet, but we may at some point. I'll pass on your best wishes, though.'

'Of course.' Dr Roshni resumes writing and smiles at both of us. 'Keep me updated.'

'Come on Chloe...'

As we walk along the corridor, Jo says, 'You look shocked.'

'I just... I don't think I could ever be a part of that. Telling a Mum there's something wrong with her baby's heart rate when there's not. Does that kind of thing happen?'

'Well, from Roshni's point of view she's keeping the ward and the women safe. It's really busy and she doesn't want to be in a situation she doesn't have time to manage. So it's not great, I agree, but keeping women and babies safe is our role as midwives too. I might have a chat to Roshni but when we have a quiet time to think. You'll learn, don't worry. You're mainly observing right now anyway.'

Now my excitement has fallen away I can feel I'm tired and hungry. My limbs are heavy. I follow Jo back into the room and smile at Bob, who's been making tea for all of us in the kitchen, and try and pull the atmosphere of the birth room back around me.

At 3am, Jo encourages Brenna to get out of the pool as her contractions are slowing down. She kind of panthers around for a bit, with a sheet wrapped around her and with Bob and me in tow. This goes on for an hour and she has some toast, which she vomits back up into a cardboard bowl and then she tells us that if we won't let her get back into the water she's getting into her car and driving home. We refill the pool.

At 4am, she's having five contractions every ten minutes and they're making her pant.

At 5.30am Brenna gives an insane, ear-wrenching scream that touches every part of me. The room smells of overheated bodies, Lucozade and fresh faeces. She has been pushing on and off for the last hour and Jo has stopped me from doing listen-ins. She's quicker. I'm just writing them down for her and plotting them on the partogram, the graph we use to track progress and the heart rate. I'm hoping against hope that I'm doing this right.

'Fuck this,' Brenna mutters, in between contractions, 'Fuck this!'

'Do you want the gas, honey?' says Bob, who's kneeling

next to her and sponging her down with a flannel from a bowl of ice.

'It doesn't fucking do anything!'

Jo smiles.

'We should really examine you again Brenna, would that be that okay?'

'In the... pool?' she's panting, on her way to contracting again. Then 'I can't do this!'

'You are doing this. You've done it before. You're doing fine,' says Jo, calmly, fishing something out of the water with a sieve and putting it in the bin.

Bob backs off from the pool as Jo puts her gloves on and I feel for him. He's watching both of us, nervous now, tall and somehow emasculated despite his overnight stubble. He grimaces at me.

'There we go... oh, it's just sat here!' Brenna screams as Jo moves her hand under the water and I wince. But Jo's grinning.

'This baby will be here really soon. Chloe, can you grab those towels? Stick them on the trolley, wheel it over and then press the buzzer for me for our second pair of hands...'

I follow her instructions and approach the pool again. There's quite a bit of bloody stuff floating around in it, which worries me, but Jo seems entirely unconcerned as she's taking her gloves off, opening sterile packs and checking the cord clamp.

'Thank you... Bob, come here, she'll need you for this bit...'

I have a brainwave and put a pillow on the floor and Bob comes and kneels on it. He closes his eyes and presses his face to Brenna's hand and my heart tugs at the gesture.

Then Brenna screams again, spit flying from her mouth, and his eyes fly open, looking like he's been electrocuted.

Jo says, 'Ah, the waters have gone,' and I can see it, an area of straw-coloured liquid has rocketed into the pool and a dark, glossy, auburn round is visible and Jo beckons me saying, 'Quick, quick, put your hands over mine –'

I do so, scrambling awkwardly, pinned to the side of the pool by Jo and she says, 'Slowly! Brenna, slowly now, listen to me, breathe the baby out!'

Brenna screams, long and hard, open-mouthed and I swear I feel my ear drums rattle as the head appears, centimetre by centimetre, ears, hair, chin and then suddenly there's a twist and the shoulders are out too, like a cork from a bottle, and my and Jo's hands bring the slick baby to the surface and into Brenna's arms.

The whole thing is over in seconds and Bob is crying and Brenna is crying and they tilt their heads to each other with their baby screaming harshly and outraged between them.

'Oh, thank fuck! Hello, hello you!' Brenna touches her baby's face, chest, hair and back, over and over. I can hear the blood rushing in my ears, my heart beating like I've just sprinted.

The baby is covered in a white creamy substance and the cord is twisted and purple, like a huge thick telephone cable disappearing under the water. The baby's eyes are open and alert, looking around, calmly at odds with the crying. The water is tinged red. This is not what many people would think of as beautiful, but the scene is gorgeous and I can't take my eyes off them.

Jo exhales behind me. 'Congratulations,' she says, 'You've got baby number three. You can cancel that buzzer, Chloe. Looks like we didn't need help after all.'

* * *

The day shift is beginning out in the corridor, but in here it's still dark, quiet and night-time. The projector is off. I think I can hear a magpie chattering in the tree outside, perhaps two of them.

Brenna is settled in the hospital bed, her eyes glittering, touching her daughter's back, bum and feet as she feeds. She's wearing a Rolling Stones t-shirt now under her dressing gown and her dark hair has gone all floppy. As I lean over to hug her goodbye, she smells like her baby; new, sweet, warm skin.

'Is there a box you can drop the ginger ones off in, Chloe, if you decide not to keep them?' says Bob.

'Shut up. You begged for another. Don't listen to Daddy, you're gorgeous,' says Brenna.

The baby's hair is a deeper red than ginger, in my opinion, an unusual colour that I haven't seen on a newborn before. Her fists are clenching and unclenching in greedy pleasure as she sucks.

'Is it okay to call her Violet if she has red hair?' Brenna asks Bob.

'It's not like she was going to be born with purple, is it? We could dye it. You want that sweetie, purple hair? Book you in for a cut and colour next week?'

I say, 'I think it's a lovely name. She's so pretty.'

'Or a wig perhaps,' says Bob. We ignore him.

'She's pretty huge,' says Brenna. Then she thanks me and I assure her I didn't do a thing.

'You kept me calm. Sorry for screaming so much. And I dread to think what a hard time you and Jo were getting outside... I know I'm a pain.'

'I'm sure that's not true.'

'Are you?' she looks me in the eye with an intelligent, searching look. 'Anyway, we'll get out of here soon. We'll get back to the kids, they'll be so confused... was it Dr Roshni out there by any chance?'

'Yeah,' I say. Bob looks uncomfortable and I wonder if he heard the conversation. I remember he was making drinks in the kitchen while it happened. *Bugger.* He looks away and I wonder what to say.

'She's a good doctor,' says Brenna, coolly, surprising me. 'I get the feeling she was thinking about her own kids when I saw her in clinic and I told her my plan. It's not something she'd ever do, but she didn't make me feel like a bad mother about it.'

'Did you...?'

'Did I..?'

'Did you feel supported?'

'I felt like she was doing the very best she could and I can't ask for more than that.' She nods, briskly. 'You have to be grateful we live in an age where maternity care is given to everyone. Expert opinions are the price we pay. I'm lucky I can cope with that kind of thing. Anyway, Chloe, go home and go to sleep.'

I'm in awe.

Jo is writing notes and getting ready to go.

'Have we scared you off, then?'

'Not yet. I'm just a bit tired. Thanks, Jo.' I'm struggling into my coat, so exhausted that I can't feel anything from my knees down, kind of like being drunk, but less fun. We walk together in companionable silence to the hospital entrance.

'I'm impressed. Your first birth! How will you celebrate?'

I smile. Everything is just beyond fantastic.

'Have breakfast when you get back, then get into bed and

don't get up again until at least midday,' she says, 'Get yourself into a routine with nights, that's what I do. You can only cope if you've got your reserve...'

She nods at me then starts walking towards the car park and says, 'Job well done!' without turning around.

6

Request

Thursday, 1st February 2001

It's one of my days off placement and Sadie and I are sat up on the second floor of McDonald's. She considered and decided against a McFlurry. You're not supposed to have soft-serve icecream in pregnancy, in case of listeriosis, which I was debating telling her about, but I don't want to be bossy. It turned out she knew already. In the end she got a big cookie and a coke and I've got a cup of tea and some chips. We're up against the big window watching the Saturday shoppers wander down the winter sunlit street.

She's perched on a stool, all decked out in a ripped shirt held together with safety pins, a mini skirt and purple arm warmers with fingerless gloves. She's thirty-two weeks now and as her bump has got more obvious, her sense of fashion has gone on the offensive. She kind of looks like a pregnant Pink.

She breaks up her cookie and tips her head back to get all the crumbs into her mouth. I take a sip of my steaming tea and put my hands around my paper cup. It's cold up here, but quiet.

'What's your Mum saying about it all now?' I ask.

'She's excited. She's told all her mates at Step. She's got dummies and feeding stuff and she buys a new babygro each time she does the shopping.'

'Are you excited?' I ask.

Sadie presses her lips together and considers.

'Most days, I'm excited, yeah. I want to meet my baby. But I'm tired of waiting. I wish I could get a job and a flat but Mum wants me to finish my GCSEs.'

She waves at her bump.

'This is a bit of a problem, y'know. No one's got jobs for me. I've tried. Didn't even make anything out of the kittens. I just ended up giving them to mates.'

'Well GCSEs are a good thing, aren't they?'

''Spose so. I'm fed up of being skint, though.'

'If you go on to college they'll give you thirty quid a week EMA.'

She makes a huffing noise.

'It's fine for you, I hate school, haven't got a clue. You always knew you wanted to be a midwife...'

'You'd be an amazing midwife...' It's not the first time she's brought this up. I want to be encouraging.

'Oh, whatever. Teen Mum.' She does the kind of eye roll where she looks capable of knocking herself out. I try to put confidence into my voice.

'No, you'd be perfect. You don't stand for any bull and you'd really care about the women.'

'Not like Karen,' she says, without dropping a beat.

'I don't think you could be like Karen if you tried.'

She shakes her head, gives me a small, wry smile and puts her hands on her belly.

'Are you still not getting on with Karen? Have you thought

about switching midwives?' I ask, but she's distracted.

'She's kicking...'

'She? So you think you know now?'

The sex of her baby and whether she can tell or not is one of her favourite subjects. We talk about it every time we meet up.

'I think it's a girl.'

'Yeah? Why?'

'Just a feeling. I get kicked a lot but it's not like I'm being booted, y'know? I think she's a she.'

'Any names picked out?'

She's drifting, watching a young woman with a baby in a polka-dot sling go past. We silently watch three more mums, flanking each other on the pavement, in winter coats and scarves. They step into a coffee shop, chatting and lifting each other's buggies over the threshold. Sadie sighs.

'You okay?'

'Yeah. Never having sex again, though, that's for sure.'

'If I had a penny for every time a midwife's heard that.'

'No. Really. I can't imagine wanting...' she trails off.

I wait. I've tried to get Sadie to talk about her ex-boyfriend before but she won't. Any questions, anything she classes as nosy and she changes the subject or goes quiet and moody.

'You seem happier with it all, anyway. You've stopped asking about booking that epidural in advance.'

'Yeah, well, whatever happens, happens. I didn't realise you could be so in charge of it. I'll try all the positions and the bath and everything... I wish it was closer to the due date, time's going so slowly.'

I eat a chip.

'You just have to be patient for this last bit.'

'*Be patient!*' she waggles her finger, imitating perhaps me and perhaps Karen and I laugh.

'Is that so bad?'

'No. Having one of these fogey midwives there during labour is going to be horrible, though, I'll hate it.'

'Hey, they might be lovely. You don't know who you'll be with yet. Odds are it won't be Karen, she works on community. If you don't like the midwife you end up with in labour, it's actually really important you swap to someone else. You can ask for that. You have to be comfortable with them, don't forget.'

'Right, like they'll listen. No one listens.'

Then she stops and looks at me. And the penny drops. I realise this is why we're here talking, why she has asked me to come out, that's she's been wanting to ask me for a long time.

'Chloe, will you look after me? I can't stand midwives always telling me what to do.'

I wonder what I can say that won't offend her.

'I mean they have to tell me if I'm doing something stupid, right, but tell me a bit nicer. What if I'm having contractions and doing really well but they start telling me off about everything and get all judgemental because I'm young?' She's staring down at the grey plastic table, tracing a circle with her finger.

I start to say 'I'd love to –' and she turns and beams at me like the sun coming up.

'Really? Chloe, that's so amazing, even if something goes wrong I'll feel –'

I hold my hands up and stop her mid-sentence. 'But I'm not sure I can.'

'Oh. Okay.' She doesn't meet my eye, just shrinks into her shirt. I feel awful. Not for the first time, I come to the conclusion that this is a girl who's been let down by a lot of people.

'I really want to. And I'm going to try. But it's part of the rules, I'll have to ask my tutors. I might have just got off shift when you go into labour, right? So I'd be too tired to be safe.'

'I'll let you know when it's starting, though, okay? I thought you said the first bit would take ages? So you'd have time to catch up on sleep before I really needed you?'

Her expression is set, like I'm trying to get out of it. I think fast.

'Well, yeah, that'd be ideal. It's often a bit unpredictable, though. But I'd love to be there. Honestly, I'm honoured you asked me. I think you'll do well. You'll be a good baby-haver.'

'Yeah? Why d'you think that?'

The expression on her face lets me know I'm on the right track so I put my hand on her arm and force myself to hold her gaze, trying to get her to cling to this certainty.

'Oh, I just do. You're young and fit and healthy and you're more concerned about who's going to be there for you rather than the pain. It's a really good attitude.'

She sits tall, wanting to believe me. I try not to smile but she looks like a pigeon puffing out her chest or something.

'Oh, right. Thanks. Well, don't put yourself out or anything. If you can't, you can't. But I wanted to ask.'

I lean back and smile at her.

'Whatever happens, remember, you get to make all of the decisions. You hold all the cards.' I think she believes me and out of everything I've done so far as an aspiring or student midwife, I think this is what I'm most proud of.

7

Personal Growth

Saturday, 3rd March 2001

I step off the bus out into the cold, crisp March morning. There's something peaceful about being on the quiet streets so early and I have that exhausted-to-the-bone, giddy triumph that comes from having survived a week of nights. I'm beyond tiredness now.

These were eight-hour shifts, much easier than twelve-hour ones, and I have a post-night routine as per Jo's instructions. I catch the hospital hopper, which takes forever but ends up nearly outside our door. Then I have a deep bath with lavender oil added to the water, stockpile calories in the form of porridge and then sleep for as long as I can before heading back into labour ward. There've been some lovely normal births, two caesareans and one emergency ventouse. It's been exhausting and a whole five days off is a heavenly thought.

I turn into our front garden and stop, sigh and hitch up my placement backpack. Helga has left me a present of a dead blackbird on the doorstep. She hasn't so much killed it as dissected and displayed it like an anatomy lesson.

Dad will still be asleep. I'm back before seven as it was

quiet and they let me go before the end of the shift. As I put my key in the door, I grin as I remember how the night began. I forget her name, but the Mum stepped over the threshold of her labour room roaring about an epidural and pushing. We had to fish her slippery, screeching baby out of her tights and I don't think I've ever seen such surprise on someone's face.

Helga chirrups and weaves around my legs as I put the kettle on.

'I'm not talking to you, murderer,' I tell her and then I go out and wrap the bird in an old *Leicester Mercury* and spray the step with bleach. Up close I can see it's not a blackbird after all, it's a starling, the feathers glossy and metallic, with a sheen of green and purple. It's a shame. Dad likes birds.

'I'm so sorry,' I find myself saying as I put it into the compost bin and replace the lid. It's slightly crazy to be talking to a dead bird, but the tiredness has got rid of all my filters, and everything I'm thinking is bubbling up to the surface, 'It's in her nature, I'm afraid. Not much I can do.'

As I come back in and I'm washing my hands, there's an enormous crash above my head which makes me jump and I slop warm water all down my front.

'Dad! What was that?!'

I reach for a tea towel, the damp patch on my uniform cooling quickly. I just want to run myself a bath and get on with my wind down. I yell again and he calls back, 'I'm fine Chlo! Just dropped something...' His tone sounds panicked.

I wait for a beat and then shout, 'But what are you doing?' No response. I mop up a bit and then stand watching the steam rising from the kettle.

There's an almost imperceptible scraping noise from above.

I creep through the kitchen to the bottom of the stairs and listen hard. I can hear cars going past. I wonder if he's carpentering again, converting the attic. It's a weird time of day for it though and my intuition, sadly honed where Dad's concerned, is nagging at me.

There are a few small bumps. I pad up the stairs and knock.

'You okay in there? I'm making porridge, d'you want some?'

A pause. Then, 'Yeah that'd be great Chlo, porridge, thanks, mmm!' He sounds desperate. I exhale.

Fuck it. I just don't want to know. It can wait until after I've slept.

I'm about to withdraw my hand, when, through dreamlike tiredness, I realise there is white light around his doorframe that far outstrips the murky morning sun. I stand and look at it.

Then, with foreboding, I push the door.

Spilling from the room is a cold light, science-fiction light, autopsy light.

Dad is staring down at me from the attic hatch.

He's wearing just his boxers and the black t-shirt he sleeps in, holding onto a ladder that rises to the attic. His head is bent because he can't straighten up in the space. It's new and well-made and smells like freshly cut wood. His expression is frozen, horrified.

Then I realise what I can smell is not wood. Behind him, I can see the outline of jagged-edged leaves and soft furry stems, the dark richness fresher than I've ever smelt it before, making me lightheaded.

I experience a dropping sensation like I'm plummeting and an unwilling drum beat starts in my chest, which moves up my spine and turns into a roar in my ears.

'Chloe. Don't worry, this is temporary, they're just going to mature and then –'

He trails off at my expression, his hands held up in defence.

I climb the ladder and he protests but I step around him, pushing him to one side of the hatch and he stumbles and almost falls. I don't care.

From the top step, I can see the whole attic room has been transformed. There are eight mature cannabis plants in large black pots and he's coated the vents with aluminium foil. A few lamps in rectangular metal cages of mesh are held in place by duct tape. There is a radiator, thermometer, a plug on a timer and a fan that ticks and whirrs, its head moving from side to side.

'*How could you?*'

'It's just for occasional use. Personal use.' He looks ridiculous, his legs are thin and white sticking out from underneath his t-shirt and this makes me even more furious.

'*Personal use?* Shut up. No, don't shut up, tell me *how you could do this in our house? In Mum's house?*'

'It's just for me, it's a Class B –'

'Where did you even get it?'

'The fans and foil are from B&Q, the wood I got from my supplier.'

'Not the fans!'

'Oh. Well, Roger introduced me to the guy with the seeds but I shouldn't tell you who, best you don't know, Chloe –'

'Oh my God. The whole thing could burst into flames! Is that why you were stealing the letters before I could get to them? The electric must be costing a fortune... holy shit. Are you stealing power? Where from?'

'It'll work out cheaper, Chloe, personal use over a year –'

'Will you stop saying that! Personal use – I'm not an idiot! Oh, maybe I am an idiot. Maybe I'm totally fucking naive!'

It's the neat competence of it all that makes me so angry.

All other adult responsibility has fallen away, but when it comes to this he's a fucking entrepreneur.

I climb back down the ladder, nearly falling in my haste, and slam the door behind me.

I go and sit at the kitchen table, in the light that's come up over the shed. I put my head in my hands and sob, terrible, tear-filled sobs. My eyes hurt. So does my chest. Everything hurts.

After a few minutes, Dad comes into the kitchen. What now? *What do I do?* He clatters around and then a cup of tea appears at my elbow. I ignore it.

'Chloe. You're not saying anything.'

'I don't know what to say.'

He edges into the room and stands across the table, behind the chair for protection as if I'm going to attack him. Well, I just might.

'Oh Chloe, don't cry. I'll start.'

'Don't you *dare.*'

I hate crying. I've done so much of it.

'How were you planning not to end up in prison?'

'Okay. Look. I got out of balance with weed at the beginning of this year, I know that. But it's a good fit for me. I know what you're going to say, but I think I would have ended up on antidepressants without it and that's so much worse. That would have been the government's choice of drug, not mine.'

He's put some jeans on. His lined, thin face and the grey in his hair is making him look so old. I can't tally him with the man who bathed me and Ali, took us to school, cooked for us for years and helped us with homework.

'I was using cannabis for sixteen hours a day or about that when it got really bad. And I had this moment of clarity when

I could see it was too much, d'you remember? I thought I couldn't cope without it... and your Mum.'

His voice wobbles.

I find a piece of tissue in my uniform pocket and wipe my face, one eye then the other, and take a ragged breath.

'Don't bring Mum into this.'

He looks at me and smiles as if I don't know what I'm saying and this makes my temper rise and it fills me like a drug itself.

'I went down to just one a day, do you remember?'

'No. I just remember you being a mess.'

'Okay. Yes, a mess, but just one spliff a day. And now that's all I do. As a social thing. This harvest will last me all year. And your uncle helped me set up the room. It's just for personal use –'

'Will you stop saying that! I'm not stupid, how much is all that worth? Are you telling me *none* of it will be sold? Oh God, I am stupid, what do I do at uni, Dad? I can't be living in a cannabis farm –'

'Chloe, will you please *listen* to me. You don't even need to know. It'll be so much better if you forget all about it. The harvest is coming up, it'll all be over and you can't get charged for something you didn't even know about.'

'But I *do* know.'

I can see the whisky bottles on top of the fridge and for a moment I'm tempted. But that's stupid. Every time I've tried to get drunk I've felt out of control and more unhappy and at this time in the morning it'd be awful. The room is already spinning. I take a big breath and try and look at this sensibly.

'I can sort of understand you needing a bit of weed to get you through the hard patches. Sort of. I can forgive that. But growing it? I'm a criminal by not turning you in. Having it in the attic... my course, everything I worked so hard for would disappear.'

I look at Dad and the red circles around his eyes and I realise he's been smoking this morning already. He's a liar. I hate him for it.

'Think about it, though. No, come on Chloe, listen. It's about our freedom. Decriminalising cannabis would mean destabilising the coke lords, the whole criminal system would fall over.'

He's sliding into his fiction, getting self-righteous. I know there's no point arguing when he's like this, but listening to it is making me cry even harder.

'It's much better I smoke something homegrown, organic and if friends get a little bit too well, then I'm doing them a favour. Some of the stuff around here kills people because of what it's cut with. Did you hear about the embalming fluid? It's crazy, they criminalised cannabis because it was a drug used by blacks in the US, it's not even as dangerous as alcohol –'

It's like I've forgotten how to breathe. I gasp for air and then say, 'Oh, so you're some kind of *activist*? A grow room in the attic and tinkering about means you're fighting for justice?'

'It's not a grow room really, not hydroponics, nothing like. It's not some big operation. It's just me and a watering can and some lamps because you can't grow it outside. Look, you don't know about these things.'

'I shouldn't be having to deal with this. I'm going to end up with one parent dead and the other in prison and a sister who doesn't give a shit.'

He steps over and tries to put his arm around me, but I push him away.

'Please don't touch me.'

As I get up I catch his expression and he looks so sad. Well, he can be. Let him be the one hurting in the real world for once.

I go up to my room and get my travel bag and start putting clothes, toiletries and books into it, while I dial on the cordless phone. I call Ali, twice, but there's no response. Then Jos. Again, nothing.

I have a dreadful, deadening sense of being totally alone and the tears cascade down my face. I dial again and the phone rings five times before he picks up.

'Hey Chloe... it's really early, how are you?'

I'm silent, unable to explain, but I know he can hear my unsteady breathing. I hear him sit straight up in bed.

My voice comes out in a plaintive bleat that I hate.

'I've just done my last night and Dad has... Christopher, Dad's done something awful. Is the offer of living at yours still on?'

'Yeah. Yeah, of course it is. Chloe, what's happening? Are you safe? He hasn't hit you, has he?'

'No, nothing like that...'

'Can you tell me over the phone?'

'I don't even know where to start.'

'What do you need me to do?'

'Can you come and pick me up? Just call me from outside in the car, don't come into the house.'

'It's okay. I'm on my way. Everything will work out, you'll see.'

I hang up. I sit for a moment and then realise I'm still in my uniform and I change into a jumper and jeans.

I pack my mobile phone charger, underwear, socks, *Mayes Midwifery*, *The Good Breastfeeding Guide*, *Spiritual Midwifery* and *Midwifery Supervision in Practice*, as well as my essay folders. My pill is in my makeup bag.

When I go back downstairs, Dad is nowhere to be seen. I feed Helga, filling her bowl with dry food, which she wolfs down.

I stroke her velvet ears and she makes a threatening noise like I'm after her crunchies. My throat tightens.

I write Dad a note. As I'm doing it, I hear a car pull up outside.

Please remember to feed Helga.
If she runs away I will _never_ forgive you.

I go out to the car as my phone starts ringing. Christopher gets out and takes my bag off me and puts it in the boot. Then he hugs me to him and I try to relax into it but I can tell this kindness is going to make me cry again and maybe not stop. There's a silence. He doesn't seem upset, but I'm worried about offending him.

I get into the front seat and he pulls out of the drive.

'I'm sorry it's under these circumstances,' I say, after a pause. 'Moving in.'

'It's okay. Chloe... what did he do? Can you tell me? He hasn't... he didn't try to –?'

I realise what he's asking and laugh, wildly and meet Christopher's grey eyes in the mirror. His concern is vice-like.

'Oh, God. No. He's not like that. No, he's just made a really big mistake.'

Silence.

'Do you want to go somewhere first? For breakfast? I don't think I've even got milk in. Shall I just stop and get some?'

'Yeah. Thanks. I mean no to breakfast out. I've been up since last night, I'm not thinking straight.'

'Anything else? Tissues? Sleeping tablets?'

'No. Thank you, though.'

He's being sweet and concerned and I can see there's a bit of him that's even enjoying it, rescuing me. He stops at Tesco and I slump down in my seat with my head in my hands while he goes in. A woman in the car next to me is shooting me glances. I must look awful. Oh, I hate this. After what seems like forever, Christopher comes out with shopping bags.

Back at his I sit at the counter and fight to stay awake. He puts away peanut butter, brown bread, fruit and dark chocolate. He offers me posh coffee, his answer to everything, which I decline. I don't think coffee could keep me awake at this stage, but the thought of being trapped in consciousness and strung out unable to sleep is terrifying. I just want to crawl into bed, but after everything he's done, I don't feel I can just disappear into his room.

The way Christopher moves around the kitchen is graceful. He has a place for everything and the kitchen surfaces are clean. The fridge is half empty and everything is in Tupperware or stacked by type, the carrots, courgettes and celery lined up. I think about Dad in his boxers. I think about Helga and my heart flares.

'We'll have to go back and get some more of your clothes and stuff, right?'

'Mmm. I'll get Ali to help. She can let me know when he's not in.'

Tears are welling up again and I wipe at them before Christopher gets his head out of the cupboard. He comes and sits next to me.

'You poor thing. Can you tell me yet? No, okay, sorry. I won't ask. We'll work out what to get in for food, what you want to eat in the evening, things that girls need...'

I blink.

'Things that girls need?'

'Oh, you know, I'm not really set up for a girl living here. Shampoo and... things.'

I laugh shakily and he smiles, not sure why he's amused me but glad anyway.

'Right. Thanks. I'm all good for that kind of stuff for now at least. And with shampoo, I'm not fussy and I can chip in money wise –'

'I know, I know. We can talk about all that. Let me look after you today, though.'

When I get into Christopher's bed the sheets are cold. He's still in the room getting his swimming stuff out of the drawer and he sees my face, throws back the covers and hops in.

'Oh my Lord. You're freezing.' He rubs my hands between his, 'Better?'

'Yeah, thanks.' I'm grateful but as he rolls me over and I lie in his warm arms, I'm desperate to be alone, to lose myself in sleep and not be thinking about any of this.

'I'm very glad you're here, you know.'

Being held feels good, but his shoulder is too bony to sleep on. I make my breathing go soft and regular and keep my eyes closed. After a few minutes he gets up, tucks his duvet and a blanket around me and closes the door.

Sleep comes over me deep and heavy, but the first few times I drop off I jerk awake again, my muscles confused at the relaxation, my brain still guarded.

As I eventually drift off and real sleep starts to beckon, one part of my brain won't turn off. Does Christopher think I'm an idiot? Does he feel pity for me? Probably. Maybe I'm too busy for Dad to tell me anything. Maybe I'm unapproachable. Perhaps if I hadn't put pressure on him to give up smoking he could have told me and we could have made it manageable somehow. Maybe I forced him into it. Or maybe I should just give up on him.

8

Fiesta

Noelia has invited us to a Spanish dinner and revision evening at her house in Bradgate. I pick up Mehreen from where she lives with her parents off Evington Road and Ada from the student halls. We drive out of the dark city and Ada sings along to *Driftwood* in her German accent, with far more cheer and force than I think Travis ever intended.

I finished placement late on Friday, after a clinic which went on way longer than planned, and I had my HCA shift this morning, so I'm strung out on exhaustion, a common theme for me, but I really need to do some preparation for this exam.

This is the first of our 'Objective Structured Clinical Examinations'. I'm finding it hard to revise at Christopher's as he needs quiet to work and me chanting about chest compressions apparently isn't helpful. Resus will definitely come up, according to the third years, but there are so many other possibilities that I'm stressing about it. The OSCE will be videoed so the tutors can watch it back and this is a pretty terrifying prospect.

As I pull up to park in the drive, Noelia is looking out of

the kitchen window and waves to us, her cheeks flushed and her curls wrapped up in a red bandana. She has a gorgeous house, with a thatched roof and willow trees surrounding it and she comes outside crunching on the gravel to wave us in (*pasar, pasar!*), past the jam jar full of cigarette butts on her doorstep, towards delicious smells of lemons and hot olive oil.

'Probably don't sit on the sofa! I have some friends who come to sew. I haven't checked for needles yet.'

In the lounge there are hand-knitted throws, a dressmaker's dummy wearing a sunhat and coloured glass lanterns on the bookcase, mantelpiece and windowsills. We go through and sit at her heavy wooden kitchen table. There are bead curtains between the rooms and the kitchen has been painted in jaunty orange and blue, which doesn't match the figure of Christ on a crucifix in a bloody crown of thorns hanging on the wall.

She sees me looking at it and says, 'Horrible, yes. But it was Mamma's. She likes to know I have it. And my father does... he's old man now, sitting in the sun, smoking. He's sad I'm not in Spain, of course. But him and my Mamma and my cousins send me cassettes in the post, they record themselves telling jokes and the news, sometimes he sings to me, he has a good voice... It's too difficult for me and Teo to go often. The flight's not expensive, but finding the time away is hard. My Mamma hates that we don't go.'

This has come out in a torrent. She wants to talk. Then she asks me about Dad and I freeze and fumble for something to say.

Ada and Mehreen are looking at me curiously. I've told Noelia a little bit over coffee, though none of the illegal stuff. It could get her into trouble as much as me. I smile, but I know I must be grim-faced because Noelia says, 'Sorry Chloe. I talk too much. My tongue has an engine. Tell me about your boy?'

'My boy?'

'Christopher. What it's like living with him?'

'Oh, you know. Men. They're all the same, aren't they? Bursting in on you when you're shaving your legs in the bath...' My stomach clenches. I don't know why I'm saying this, it implies Christopher is doing something wrong. He's even put a lock on that door now, after I asked.

I'm paying half rent (and I had to fight for that, but paying nothing at all is too weird); I keep up with the washing and iron his shirts, but he buys mostly organic and does almost all of the cooking, admittedly because I don't know where things go back in the cupboard, but still. And he's not mentioned my midwifery future, Dad or anything else I don't want to discuss since that first morning. He lets me curl up on the sofa with my textbooks and insists on doing the washing up after dinner. It makes me feel guilty, as he works as hard as me.

But I am getting more sleep since moving in, which I'm very glad of, and my dreams are more settled, which since Mum died has always been a good measure of how I'm coping. I went through a phase of having to kill her in my dreams in the first year. Over and over, hit her with the car, drown her, stab her. I'm so grateful those are gone now.

As Noelia finishes cooking, we all start playing 'midwifery ring buzz' at the tiny kitchen table. This involves Ada asking us questions from her stack of meticulous, blue-penned revision cards and the rest of us shouting out facts and figures, trying to beat each other. I'm flushed with happiness. What a nerd.

'Okay, everyone, sterile technique for catheterisation. Tell me the steps.'

We're making an immense amount of noise and talking over each other, shouting about consent. Mehreen is saying 'Chloe gets five points for knowing saline is just as good as antiseptic,' but no one's listening, when a door I had assumed was a kitchen cupboard, but apparently has stairs behind it, opens and we all jump.

'Evening, ladies.'

It's a young guy, with an accent that's pure Leicester. He has darker skin than Noelia. We all shut up and I'm very aware we've been shouting about bladders, bowels and vaginal examinations.

I'm startled as he says something to his mother in Spanish; it's like hearing another soul pop out. I can see Noelia's bone structure in his face, sharp and mischievous, but with thinner cheeks. He has her golden-brown eyes, like dark pools of honey. We all say hello.

'Are you eating with us, Teo?'

'Nah, I'll keep working Mamma, that okay?' His eyes drift to the table where we've spread out our notes, diagrams of breasts, fetal skull sutures and worse.

Noelia nods. She's hovering over an enormous red saucepan with a slotted spoon, frying something breadcrumbed and cylindrical in batches and draining them onto kitchen roll. They smell amazing.

I watch as with concentration Teo piles these onto a plate in Jenga style, almost to the point of overflow. Then he carves off a doorstep slice of dark, dense bread, fills a tiny ceramic blue and silver bowl with olive oil and a few drops of vinegar and loads up on salad too. For a little guy, this is a lot of food.

He looks at me and grins and I realise I'm staring.

'What are they? The fried things?' I ask, to cover my confusion.

'*Croquetas*. In Spain, they make them with ham or bacon, but Mamma makes them with pumpkins and mushrooms. Cheaper and better.' He passes one to me and I bite into it.

'Wow,' I say and he laughs and puts his plates on a tray.

'You're not having the tortilla? You don't like it?'

'I'm vegan. No eggs.'

'Oh.'

Teo smiles at me and I blush. It's hot in the kitchen and I'm relieved when he disappears upstairs again.

We start eating. The basil is sweet, the tomatoes are fresh and ripe and everything is drenched in olive oil. Noelia passes us thick wedges of white and nutty-tasting cheese with a black wax rim and some kind of thick red paste to go with it. It's quince jelly, made from the fruit in *The Owl and the Pussycat*, and it's sweet and astringent.

I say, 'This is so amazing Noelia,' and everyone agrees. She tells us she's always nervous inviting people round and never tells them she's vegetarian in advance, just in case.

'But they always like the food, in the end. Meat is so heavy, I think people don't realise that flavour comes from the herbs and garlic and things like that.'

Ada asks, 'Does Teo live with you?'

'Yeah. He'll stay with Mamma until he's married. He's a good boy but he'll be watching *Top Gear* and drinking *cerveza* up there, whoever heard of studying during dinner?'

'Fair enough,' says Ada, 'Most boys don't want to talk about midwifery in detail. Or at all.'

'No, no! He's not like that. He helps me with the revision and he reads through my essays. It's great, he's a good student and he's not embarrassed.'

'Easy as that,' I say.

We're trying not to get grease on the revision cards and this time we're focusing on breastfeeding. Positioning and attachment are topics that might come up, as are all the antibodies. There are so many reasons breastfeeding is invaluable: the tiny amounts of hormones and chemicals will trigger changes that knit into a baby's immune system, benefiting them even when they're adults.

Ada asks me, 'What's the main hormone involved in the let-down reflex? Chloe?'

Looking through into the kitchen, I can see Teo has crept down the stairs again and is loading up his plates for a second round. Then he opens the fridge and takes out what is clearly a cold rice pudding.

'Chloe?'

I wonder how Noelia has made this vegan.

Teo cuts himself a huge square portion of the rice and levers it out and into a bowl. Then he opens the cupboard and adds a handful of raisins, and sprinkles cinnamon, from a height. This makes me smile; he looks so serious, like the configuration of his pudding will have a major impact on worldwide politics or the future of humanity.

In the soft light coming from the stairs and with the overhead kitchen bulb off, he is almost glowing. He turns and sees me watching him through the pink bead curtain and smiles and puts his finger to his lips. My stomach swoops in a way which is so physical that I almost think if I had my hand on my skin, I would have felt it flip over.

As he goes up the stairs again I am a bit freaked out. What's wrong with me? Christopher's amazing. And this is Noelia's son. This is *not* okay.

'Chloe? The let-down reflex?' Ada repeats the question, this time impatient.

'Sorry,' I say, 'Oxytocin. That's the hormone. Oxytocin.'

* * *

Monday, 5th March 2001

I'm working with Diane in triage and she's pretty tough. She's a very quiet woman, fifty or so with beautiful braids and an experienced manner. She gets a lot done without seeming to. You turn back and she's admitted three women and is waiting patiently for you to get the last on to the CTG.

Triage is fun, if stressful. Women come in to be assessed and then you have to work out if they need to stay and where they need to go: labour ward, the birth centre, the antenatal ward. It's an exercise in getting it all done fast. I wonder if Mum enjoyed it, or whether it was her worst nightmare because you can't get to know the women.

Diane tells me to go in with Fatima, who may or may not have pre-eclampsia and has arrived contracting hard, making a lot of noise. Her mother-in-law is with her in the corner, wearing a turquoise sari covered in little glittering mirrors that reflect spots of light onto the wall. When I smile at her, she grins at me and I see she has no teeth. I say hello but I don't think she speaks any English.

'Fatima, can I do a palpation?'

Diane is through the curtain and talking to the woman in the next bed about whether or not her vaginal discharge on the pad is green. I pull the curtain around us a bit more, which doesn't help block the sound, but it's all I can do. Fatima finishes having her contraction and looks at me wordlessly.

'Would that be okay? To have a feel of baby first, so I can do a listen in?' Fatima pulls her *shalwar kameez* up to reveal her bump. I try and work out where the baby's back is by sweeping my hands down her abdomen, following a line of soft downy hair. I'm going as fast as I can, but carefully too. I feel the baby roll under my hands, in protest at being touched, and I smile.

I can't work out much; I know I have a long way to go with this skill. It used to feel like having my hands on a lumpy pillow wearing oven mitts, but now I am beginning to feel things. I hardly ever get the easy ones, it seems, where the baby is lying head down with its back neatly tucked in, but if I had to guess, I'd say the back was on the right.

I put my fingertips over the baby's head down in Fatima's pelvis. It's a hard roundness. I catch Fatima's eye. Some midwives and obstetricians do this bit the old-fashioned way: they use one hand to grip whichever bit of the baby is down in the pelvis, but this is uncomfortable for the woman. Using both hands and moving gently is far better.

'Is this okay? You comfy?' she nods, watching me. I can barely feel any of the baby's head, it must be really low. Or I'm rubbish at this.

I sigh. I'm pretty sure this baby is head down, but I haven't got a clue where its back is.

'I think I'm going to have to get Diane to repeat the palpation, is that okay?'

Fatima nods. 'Can I have something for the pain?'

I nod, wondering how quickly I can arrange it. This is the other hard thing about triage; you only have a few minutes to sort everyone out. I feel guilty that I can't do this faster for Fatima. The skin of her abdomen starts to tighten and she starts to cry out again. Her mother-in-law is still smiling, at least.

I pop my head around the curtain. Diane is sitting at the desk, her gaze flicking between the computer and a woman's notes.

'Fatima's hurting. Can she breathe some gas after I've put the monitor on?'

'Yes. There's a canister in the third cubicle, you can take

that,' she says. 'Maybe explain she can't get hooked on it if it's early in her labour though. Hurry up, please, Chloe. In a minute I need you to go to postnatal, there's a baby who's bottle-feeding who's a bit sleepy, can you go and help? Get that feed done, then you can come back here.'

I go back to Fatima, taking the blue entonox canister with me. I wait until her contraction stops and then put the elastic straps under her back, turn on the CTG monitor and put some gel onto one of the transducers. It rattles and roars, picking up interference until I find the heart rate, on the bottom right side of Fatima's belly. I secure the straps in place.

The paper starts to feed out, tracing the baby's heart rate between 130 and 150 beats per minute, a rocky line with tiny mountains, like this baby's traversing them to get to the outside. But there's no time to get romantic. Fatima's contracting again and I open a plastic wrapped mouthpiece and attach it to the piping that comes from the canister.

Fatima knows exactly what to do. She grabs it from me and starts to inhale, holding it between her teeth.

'I think Diane's going to come and do an examination Fatima, to see how far you are. She says if you're just starting in labour we might have to rethink the gas,' I say. Her breath is drawing through the device, making a wheezing sound.

'Just during the contractions, yeah? You'll get dizzy if you do it in between.'

Fatima nods, closes her eyes and keeps breathing. I hope it's all okay.

I head to the postnatal ward and am directed towards a middle-aged mum who's trying to get her tiny 36-weeker to wake up and feed. He's jaundiced, yellow and in a maroon babygro. After a lot of persuasion, tickling his feet and cheeks, we get him to take 10ml or so, which I have a horrible feeling we'll be seeing again. But he's had something.

The postnatal midwife sees me and thanks me, and when I'm leaving calls after me, 'No, don't leave me! Labour ward might be more interesting, but we've got the Quality Street!' I giggle and keep walking.

Back in the triage room, Fatima's making even more noise than before. I pop around the curtain and watch as she finishes her contraction. On the CTG feedout, you can see from the pressure sensor I attached to the top of her bump that her contractions have been drawn as big craggy shapes, about four every ten minutes and they go on for about a minute each. It looks like proper labour to me. Someone's stopped the monitoring for now and prepared her for a vaginal examination, her trousers folded neatly in her mother-in-law's lap and a sheet over her lower half.

'Hey,' I say softly, 'How's it going?'

She opens her eyes.

'Yeah, it's okay with the gas. The doctor's going to come round, my blood pressure's only slightly up. Apparently. D'you know where the midwife is?'

'She's just in with one other lady. Then she'll be back,' I want to ask something, but I'm nervous and unsure it's the right thing to do. But you have to start somewhere.

I can see my placement backpack through the gap in the bottom of the curtain and I know my pinard is in there.

I quickly explain to Fatima that I'm a student and I might not be able to hear anything using a pinard, but I'm learning to use one and could I have a go. She asks me what a pinard is and I tell her I can show her and when I come back round the curtain with it and say it's an old-fashioned way of listening to babies, she nods, yes, I can try.

I've read about pinards a lot by now. I position the large end of it on her flank, where I'm imagining her baby's back to be and put my ear to it, trying to listen. I strain but I can't hear anything.

I'm turned towards the curtain and I see Diane come in. She frowns and I'm crestfallen because I think she's upset with me, so I stop and back away with the pinard in my hand. But she comes and takes it from me. Then she feels Fatima's baby again, who I can see is wriggling. Diane repositions the pinard and after listening and smiling for a moment, she beckons me and we swap places.

She laughs softly.

'Chloe, you're concentrating so hard that you look like you're trying to grow a new ear.' I take my hands away and balance. And then I hear it.

It's magic. A tiny, magic spell. It sounds just like the click button in a jam jar lid being depressed and released. I feel like it's the first time I've ever heard a fetal heart. Which of course, in some ways, it is. This is the real deal; it's so much more exciting than the electronic version. I listen for ten seconds or so and then Fatima starts to contract again, her skin going taught.

'Ok, Chloe, leave be,' says Diane, tugging at my shoulder, and I straighten up.

'That's so amazing. Thank you.'

'It's something we should all be doing but there's never any time. As a student, keep going, any opportunity. Most mums quite like it. Are you going to do this examination? Have you asked Fatima?'

'Um...' Fatima looks at me, glassy-eyed from the gas, and I explain, 'The vaginal examination is to see how dilated you are, did you want one? Have you discussed it already?'

She takes two more big puffs and says, 'You can do it.'

'Really?' I'm astonished. Maybe she's high on the gas.

'Um,' I say, about to thank her, but Diane pushes me towards the sink.

'Come on then, Chloe. Wash your hands. Gloves on.'

As I'm getting ready I hear Diane say, 'It's mild pre-eclampsia if anything, Fatima. It may be you don't have it, your bloods are normal. If you do have it, to explain, it's a reaction to the pregnancy, like an immune response, which causes lots of symptoms including high blood pressure. But we'll see what the doctors say. It might be this baby arrives before you have to cope with it in any case, and delivery is the best form of treatment.' Her tone is precise and reassuring.

'I don't think I understand...'

As I listen, I put the gloves on with sterile technique.

Diane is still explaining. 'It's a disease that comes only in pregnancy. It's an immune response that causes the placenta not to be 'plumbed in' and this causes your body to react in a certain way.'

'Ok. Can you tell my husband when he arrives? I can't concentrate...'

'Of course.'

Diane sees I'm ready and squeezes some sterile lubricant onto my fingers.

I've been present at a lot of vaginal examinations and I know how to do a visual inspection. Diane lifts the sheet up for me and everything looks normal, as far as I can tell. Fatima's feet are together, her legs bent at the knees. I look at Diane for reassurance and she nods.

'Tell me to stop at any time,' I say, 'I'll try and work out how dilated you are.'

When I first put my index and middle fingers in and feel around, I panic. It's like warm mud. I can't distinguish anything at all.

'I think you need to go in a bit further,' Diane murmurs. I do so and Fatima sucks the gas harder.

'Sorry...' I say, but I can feel something. There's a thin rim of something hard and as I sweep my fingers upwards, I can tell it's circular thin muscle. It's under tension. It's her cervix. *I'm feeling a cervix!* And then I move my fingers to the right and I can feel something hard and bony where the cervix has opened up and Diane asks me what I'm feeling and I say, 'I think I can feel the head! Fatima, I think your baby has hair!' and I'm not sure what Fatima's mother-in-law thinks is going on, but she cackles at me and Diane smiles.

'Can you tell how dilated the cervix is?' I move my fingers around again and Fatima starts to breathe in and out too fast, I'm causing her pain, so I remove my hand.

'This is my first VE. But I'd say it was about, um, five centimetres?'

Diane is already putting her gloves on and she repeats the examination, turning her head towards the ceiling and closing her eyes to concentrate. It takes her about five seconds and then she stops and Fatima relaxes.

'Chloe's quite right, Fatima. Five centimetres.'

I'm elated. All those hours practising with models must have paid off.

Diane turns to me, 'Shall we find Fatima a midwife who can stay with her?'

We work quickly together, gathering notes and results. Diane calls the co-ordinator to find a spare room and I help Fatima get her trousers back on.

'That's so amazing,' I keep saying.

I walk with Fatima down the corridor. We take our time, I rub her back during her contractions. I help her get settled, dim the lights and put her back on the monitor, as I've been asked to. I find a birth ball that she can use and she settles onto it gratefully.

Before I leave, I thank her once again. I look at her, unsure if she's annoyed with me for doing the examination, or scared about her labour, or what. I wish I could read her mind.

But as her husband enters the room, a tall, thin man with an alarmed expression, she says, 'It's okay, Neel. You can ask them questions, but it'll all be okay.'

Just another routine day for a first-year student midwife.

9

Fight

'God, it's chilly,' says Christopher, in just his dressing gown, heading towards the coffee machine. 'Are you okay? You look tired. And you're in your posh skirt, why?'

The weather has gone wintry, it's very cold and blowy. It's one of the days that Christopher and I can set off together for our respective campuses, as I'm not on placement. Usually, I'd take things at a leisurely pace, with Radio 1 on, maybe flicking through my lecture notes as we chat and have toast. But this morning I'm nervous because I need to persuade my tutor to let me be on call for Sadie. The thought of potentially having to tell her that I'm not allowed and she'll need to brave things on her own is making me feel dreadful.

I explain all this. Christopher frowns.

'I don't know if it sounds like such a good idea, Chloe. Shouldn't you just hope you're on when she comes in?' My stomach tenses. 'You are allowed to say no to things.'

'I know. I'd like to be there for her, though.'

'You're working six days a week already.'

'I'm coping. She's only sixteen and she really needs

someone.'

'You're only nineteen.'

'But I'm old for my age, wise beyond my years, and generally very impressive, don't you think?' I smile, but Christopher doesn't. He passes me a steaming espresso cup and I thank him and stir in some sugar as he spreads marmalade onto his toast.

'Why's she your responsibility?'

'She's not... she's just young and scared and she trusts me.'

'Mmm. I bet your lecturers are thrilled.'

I consider and swallow a mouthful of coffee, my head on one side.

'D'you think they will be? I don't know. Rosie's my personal tutor and I mean, she's really highly respected. She's the one with dreadlocks...'

Christopher makes a face.

'She knows her own mind is what I'm saying. I think she's more likely to say yes than any of the other tutors... but they might have rules about being on call and potentially missing placement.'

'Are you supposed to be looking after your friends?'

'My Mum would have said you should look after every woman like she's a friend. And anyway, I'm not looking after her as a student midwife, I'm being there as a birth partner.'

'Are you not having breakfast?'

'I'm not hungry.'

'You should have something.'

He plods off to get dressed and I wash the breakfast things and put his plate away. I can't face eating, but I put a cereal bar into the pocket of my bag.

We lock up and head into the drizzle, which has made the pavement slick and shiny, and as I take Christopher's hand, I try to forget about my meeting. I glance at him; he's expressionless. I try not to think about his reaction either. Sometimes I think I spend my whole life trying to stop thinking about things that then fight their way back into my brain and dance for attention.

There's going to be a new bookshop on Narborough Road, I force myself to notice, wedged between the Hong Kong fish and chip place and a Polish corner shop that sells really good sourdough bread. This is good. I miss normal reading, the non-midwifery kind. I can pop in and get something.

'Chloe?'

I realise Christopher's been telling me something about his PhD.

'Sorry, what?'

'I'm really careful with my time. If I treated each research participant like a friend I'd never get anything done. Especially when they're addicts, they can drag you down. You need to watch that, you'll burn out.'

'Oh that's right, I was reading those books on your desk. The stuff about chemical hooks that are there for some people and not others was fascinating...'

'Well, that's part of it. It *is* interesting, it *is* motivating, but I have to manage my time if I want to make any headway.'

We're walking fast, my arm through his, dodging shift workers on their way back from nights.

'With Sadie, it isn't about work though,' I say, 'It's about being there for her. Some of these teenagers get shoved through the system and it's just easier to shut them up with an epidural...'

'You've got enough going on with your Dad and your sister. And she's just one girl.'

'I barely see Dad and Ali at the moment.' Immediately,

I start to worry about them both. Ali texts me occasionally and I've gone over a few times when I know Dad's at his woodwork class. Helga's bowl has always been full to the point of overflowing. She's hardly going to run away.

It occurs to me that what Christopher really means is that he wants me there for him and no one else. But I shake the thought away, I don't know if that's true. It's unfair to think it.

'If no one was there for Sadie that would break my heart. She's so… innocent.'

'She can't be *that* innocent if she's got herself pregnant at sixteen.'

I look at him sideways, neat and pale in his shirt, so calm, so sure of himself.

'What the –'

He's not listening.

'And she can choose an epidural if she wants. You're always going on about choice, right? What's the big deal?'

'We'll have to wait and see, but I just don't think she'll choose an epidural if she's looked after right. I know her, we've talked about it.'

'But what you're saying is that the best choice is to go through the most painful event of a woman's life with no drugs.'

'I'm not saying that at all. And some women don't find it painful.'

'Yeah, but rarely. That's just what the feminists say, isn't it?'

'Feminists are all different. I was reading this great book the other day about how feminism doesn't know how to deal with motherhood. It struggles with women wanting to be mothers or finding empowerment in labour –'

'Yeah, so it's just the National Childbirth Trust weirdos and midwives who want to see women in pain, that's what you're saying.'

I'm stunned. I can't get my thoughts into words. I know he's wrong, but he's so much more eloquent than I am and my blood rushes, this time not in the good way that I associate with Christopher. I don't want this to be a fight, especially as we're approaching the university. I can hear the gospel choir finishing off one of their early morning practices with *Oh Happy Day* as we approach The Newarke. Even through the closed window it's loud and distracting and I can't think. I try to explain.

'If she's looked after properly I think she'll discover how good a mum she can be. Teenagers are better parents than people give them credit for. That's what I'm in midwifery for. I think I can help her.'

He sighs.

'Chloe, don't take the weight of the world on your shoulders. There's only so much you can do with someone from that background.'

His words are like a slap and I drop his hand. We're just outside the Hawthorne building and I can see Noelia across the road. I don't know whether to storm off or shout at him.

'Oh, don't have a fit. I'm sorry, okay? I didn't mean it that way. I've got a long day coming up and I'm just worried you're taking on too much.'

Before I can respond Noelia comes up to us, her long boots clacking on the pavement.

Christopher greets her, gives me a firm kiss on the cheek and says, 'Good luck. See you tonight,' and walks on towards his campus without waiting for me to respond. I watch him go and Noelia, with uncharacteristic tact, doesn't ask me what's going on.

* * *

I'm drifting, in the lecture room with its warm heaters, staring at the ceiling and listening to the desolate whine of the overhead projector. The morning lecture is on Harvard referencing. There are a lot of examples that Rosie's talking us through, her dreads twisted and pinned on top of her head. I can't imagine her in uniform. I wonder if she has to take her piercings out for work. She has multiple studs in her ears, one in her nose and a tiny silver ring in her lip, which I think is new. This morning she looks kind of like I'd imagine Medusa would if her snakes were so bored they'd fallen asleep.

I keep thinking about how I'm going to ask her. Should I talk about it as a learning thing? Or as Sadie wanting and needing me there? Why does it matter what everyone thinks? Why does Christopher have to have an opinion? I look around. Noelia is yawning and other students are slumped with their hands propping them up.

Suddenly, Rosie bangs the table in front of her with a fist and we all jump.

'Oh, my God, you lot! You can look this up. Just get your referencing right if you want your marks on your essays. Let's talk about something *interesting* instead.'

She stands up, grabbing the acetate from the projector. She's wearing Doc Martens and a black coat with little chains hanging off it, which swing as she moves. I really wonder how she gets away with dressing like that.

'Look, this third paper on the list, it's on CTGs. Why do some units use them more than others? Especially as we know they don't prevent babies dying?'

There's a silence. Then a blonde middle-aged student with a grey cardigan and a tartan scarf puts her hand up.

'Catherine. Yes.'

'Well, I thought the information about referencing was useful, but we can read it I'm sure, in our own time. I'm happy to debate.' She sounds entirely unhappy, and not that surprised. 'If you use CTGs, you don't have to listen in with a sonicaid. And then you get a print-out so you don't miss anything about the fetal heart. And you can prove it, it's there on paper, you can audit care afterwards. I don't know if your evidence is correct, it seems silly not to watch a fetal heart if you've got concerns.'

'Okay, good point,' says Rosie, nodding, 'But what if the evidence shows an experienced midwife with a pinard is safer than a CTG?'

'Wouldn't that be nice, a pinard!' Catherine giggles and I vow to use mine as much as possible next placement. 'Of course we all want to be with women for that length of time and learn that skill, but it's so manic you just have to concentrate on safety. I just don't think you know what it's like right now, Rosie.'

Rosie smiles, wryly.

'So you're saying if it's busy, we need machines to help us keep up and that leads to safer care?'

'Yeah. I saw a TV programme about American obstetrics where they had a labour ward and the monitors were hooked up to a big computer so the coordinator could see the fetal hearts all the time. Then the most experienced midwife could keep an eye on everything, everyone could benefit from her experience. Perfect.'

Noelia makes a loud and very Spanish-sounding tutting noise.

Rosie looks over at us and says, 'What are your thoughts, Noelia?'

'We should never replace care with CTGs. If there aren't enough midwives, that's a problem: we should get in touch with the union. When I was in labour I was seventeen and if I'd have been staring at a machine with no midwife in the room, I would have been terrified. I needed a role model, not a robot.'

I nudge her and whisper, 'I didn't know you were seventeen when you had Teo...'

She nods, about to say something else, but Catherine replies.

'We weren't talking about replacing midwives with machines, we were talking about whether or not CTGs have a place. You have to think about time management too. And what's more, I'm not sure women have a right to decline advice if it means we can't look after everyone else on the labour ward as well.'

'What do you mean exactly?' asks Rosie.

'Well say a really obese woman with a heart condition wants to use the birth pool. This happened a few days ago on placement and it was just ridiculous. It takes ages to sort out, you have to get the doctors in and if something goes wrong, which, let's face it, it almost always does, and they pass out you could end up really hurting your back getting them out of the water.'

I remember Brenna.

'Okay, but do you think that's the woman's right? To choose the pool against guidance?'

'If it takes staff away from other situations I don't think it's their right, no. I think it's selfish.'

'It *is* their right,' I hear myself say. 'When a woman chooses to use the pool, it's just water, but what's she's really choosing is to not be monitored on the bed, to decline intervention, to believe in her body. A waterbirth increases the likelihood of things being straightforward.'

I hadn't planned on joining in with this, but now I've started I can't seem to stop, 'She has to make the right, best decisions for her. We just have to have faith in her choice and hold space for her.'

Catherine tosses her head and smiles.

'"Hold space". I love how you young ones are.'

'What do you mean?'

'Well, some of us still have to be idealistic, I suppose.'

'I don't think high standards are idealistic...'

'No really. I love it. It's a good thing. You hold on to that,' she says. The condescension in her tone makes me clench my fists.

'Okay,' says Rosie, 'Let's keep things friendly. You're hitting on the main difficulty, the balance between informed consent and using the resources we have. But choice is paramount... midwives have always supported women with choices that doctors or 'the system' or 'society' find difficult. Right back to Plato, for instance, we know that midwives were capable of inducing abortion. It's about bodily autonomy.'

This is interesting, but I can't really concentrate. I'm ashamed of my outburst. Christopher has got under my skin.

'We have to manage the resources too. It's about the bigger picture,' Catherine says and I shrug. With calm maturity, she goes on about rising birth rates and obstetricians and the class is listening. I want to scream. Rosie is biting her lip over her piercing.

I just let Catherine talk. I've lost my nerve. But I sit with my guts twisting in anger on behalf of Sadie and all the other women who are knocked down and pushed through a system.

We break for coffee and I head to Rosie's office. I'm still not hungry at all.

* * *

As I knock I try to smile. I want to come across as calm and responsible and not at all like I'm a combination of furious and frightened, with my heart in my mouth.

'Come in!'

I manage to get to Rosie's desk without knocking over any of the towering piles of paper and sit down across from her. There are three computers and desks wedged into this tiny rectangular room. It's messy, with pens and folders everywhere, and it smells of apple cores and pencil shavings.

After a second Rosie stops typing and smiles at me. Up close, she has fine lines around her eyes. She isn't wearing any makeup and if it wasn't for her dreads, her piercings and her energy she'd look far older.

'Chloe. You're one of mine, aren't you, but we've not caught up much. How d'you get on with your OSCE?'

'Um, okay, I think. Blood pressures and venipuncture are nice topics to come up, I was happy. But you just have to see, don't you?'

'You do. But I'm sure you'll be fine, these first ones are to slide you in anyway, it's the ones at the end of this year you'll really have to perform for... Well, it's nice to meet you properly. You're a bit quiet in lectures sometimes, aren't you? But everything you've brought up has been interesting. Today was good.'

'Thanks.'

I swallow. Then I ask,

'You were away at a conference, weren't you, in Holland for a week? What was it on?'

'My research is on you lot, actually. It's on how midwives react as they qualify and develop. It's loads of fun, I get to talk to so many people.'

'Like the Dutch midwives?'

'Yeah, exactly. They're autonomous. And politically aware. Don't let me get too off topic though, I do that!' She laughs. 'What can I do for you, Chloe? Is this about what just happened? The debate?'

'Oh, no. That's all fine, it just gets heated.'

'With midwives? Yeah. Lots of different opinions. It's not like studying English or Philosophy or something. Though there are bits of philosophy involved... what we believe has an instant impact on women's lives, right?

'Um, yes. Speaking of which. What I'm really here about is I have this friend...'

'Oh yes?'

'She's pregnant and she's sixteen.' Rosie raises her eyebrows and grins.

'How's she getting on?'

'Well, she had dramas to begin with but we're all sorted now. I met her when I was volunteering at an antenatal class and we meet up for coffee sometimes. It's nice to give her a bit of support. I'm not sure her mum is coping that well. I think if it'd been last year she would have got in with a teen pregnancy midwife, but you know how it is.'

'I do know. Who's her midwife?'

'Karen Hodgson.'

'And she hasn't clicked?' she asks, shrewdly, settling in her chair.

'No,' I answer, unsure of how much to say, 'She asked me if I could look after her and I said I didn't know... I'd happily settle for being her birth partner, though. She wants someone she knows there.'

I look out of the window and watch the black silhouette of

a bird in the white foggy sky and try to find the right words to describe how important this is, without saying what I think of Karen. I open my mouth to speak again but Rosie interrupts me.

'Well, I'm not sure you can care for her at your stage, as a first year,' she says, and my heart plummets. 'Mostly what you're doing right now is observing. But you can be with her. You can be on call and everything.'

'I can?' this comes out much higher-pitched than I'd intended.

'You can. You've got a mobile phone? And transport? Great. Just make sure you're there in an unofficial way. Don't get involved in anyone else's care. Remind the midwife that you're a birth partner and you shouldn't be called out of the room. And stand your ground, right?'

Rosie checks her watch. It has tiny black stars on a silver face. 'We should head back in. If anyone gives you any trouble about this, tell them I approved it.' I'm beaming.

As we move towards the door it's pushed open and Rosie sighs and sits down again in the manner of someone who's been held up in this way far too many times. It's Enid, balancing a stack of folders and a mug of tea. We wait for her to move past and she slides down the gap in the desks with practised grace and arranges herself in her chair. She takes us both in and frowns.

'Such a squeeze. Morning, you two. Chloe Cawthorne, what are you doing in here?'

I say good morning, and I'm about to tell her but Rosie gets there first.

'I've just approved Chloe being a birth partner for a friend of hers, Enid.'

Enid looks down at her paperwork, uncaps her pen and

says 'Oh.'

I look at Rosie, unsure how to react. Enid goes on, 'Have you told her yet, this friend?'

'No. I was going to today though.'

'Mmm. Well, I'd think very carefully about that decision, if I were you. Be certain before you commit.'

'It's great practice for Chloe being with a woman though, right?' Rosie puts one hand on my shoulder and squeezes it and I feel a bit better.

'Who's the client?' Enid asks.

'I met her at the Aylestone antenatal class,' I venture. 'You were there the day she turned up, actually.'

'Oh yes. One of Karen's ladies, was it? And she's latched on to you. I see. Was she a teenager? Just think hard about what it means. Being on-call is very challenging, especially around your commitments. It's hard to say no, but being there for friends and family is complicated. What if something goes wrong?'

The way she says it, it's a throwaway comment, a useful piece of advice from someone with experience. But my heart is racing.

'Enid, we're late for our lecture.'

'Alright! Best of luck Chloe. Think about what I said though.' She waves her hand at us regally.

As we walk back downstairs together Rosie says, 'Enid's been doing midwifery for so long that she's kind of matter-of-fact about it all. But she's an amazing midwife to have around. And she really cares. Exactly who you want to see on the horizon when you've got an emergency.'

'Oh, I know. I think a lot of her,' I say.

There's a silence. We're reflected as we walk towards the big glass double doors. Rosie is all decked out in black and I'm in my denim jacket, my skirt with the little purple flowers and my ballet flats. We couldn't look more different.

'Enid and I totally disagree about some things. I think caring for your friend will teach you loads. And as for on-call, you're young, fit and healthy. You'll cope with the lack of sleep.'

'I think so too.'

'Good,' she says. 'Right. We're going to look at the Nursing and Midwifery Code and how to use it in complex ethical dilemmas next. Let's see if we can keep ourselves out of trouble until lunch at least.'

10

Sadie's Birth

Tuesday, 10th April 2001

I'm dreaming about a nightclub which is lit with blue phototherapy bulbs. No one will let me go home despite the fact I'm so exhausted that I'm swaying. There's a baby in an incubator, yellow with jaundice. His mother is sitting beside him in a tight sequined dress over her postnatal bump and dark makeup. I ask her if she wants a drink but she just stares at me.

Christopher is behind me and he says, 'Leave her.' I say, 'But why is she ignoring me?'

The woman gets up and disappears into the crowd. I'm left to look after her baby, standing out in my uniform, among the dancers. I'm worried because I don't know how to feed the baby and I can't find my mentor anywhere in the crowd.

Christopher nudges me in the back. I groan. I want to go home.

'What is it?'

I've worked nearly forty hours in three days and my brain hurts.

'*What?*'

He nudges me again.

'Your phone.'

'Wha –? Oh.' The ringtone is jaunty and annoying and cuts into my head as reality floods through the layers of sleep. I look at the screen and it's 2.30am. Enid is right, being on call is a stupid idea.

'Sadie?'

On the end of the line, there's some muffled breathing and then a whimper.

'Hello?'

'Can I go to the hospital yet?' she says in a small voice. I sit up in bed and put a hand to my head.

'How's it going?'

'It hurts...'

We agree I'll start getting my stuff together to cycle to Dad's, as the car is there. She'll call the labour ward before confirming with me that she's on the way in, but it sounds like she's having a full-on contraction every few minutes.

I put on my brown cords, converse trainers, a blue top and my wool jumper in the dark, trying to be quiet and not wake Christopher again, and find my placement backpack. It's horribly cold in the flat. I make instant coffee so strong that a spoon would stand up in it and I sit at the breakfast bar, drunk on tiredness. The phone rings again and it's Sadie's mum, whom I've never spoken to myself before, but she sounds calm and quiet.

I go back into the bedroom and kiss Christopher goodbye. He calls me mental and rolls over to go back to sleep.

I pedal through town. It's cold enough to make my eyes water and chest ache and there's hardly anyone about. The wind cuts straight through my coat, the crescent moon and stars above me clear in that way that feels like the earth has no atmosphere and the freezing cold is falling in straight from space. But as I get close to Lincoln Street my fingers and toes get warmer, my brain wakes up and fatigue pumps adrenaline around me along with the coffee and I get my first flutterings of excitement, about being a birth partner for the first time.

The lounge light is on at home but I don't knock on the door. They're playing music and I can see the shadows of at least four people on the curtain. I can smell the weed from outside. I lock my bike in the alley and get into the car.

It isn't too busy: five women are on the board and the corridor is clear of staff. Everyone is one-to-one in rooms.

Sadie has been admitted. I peer at her details and I'm elated to see she's six centimetres dilated already. 'Nice one lady,' I mutter.

After a brief kerfuffle with the co-ordinator, who doesn't recognise me out of uniform, I walk down to the birth room.

Sadie is kneeling with her arms crossed over the Swiss ball, wearing a tiny black crop top and blue gingham bottoms. In the half-light, her body looks healthy and capable. Her mum is kneeling next to her and I join them on the mat.

'It all slowed down when we came in,' she says, 'But I think it's going again. She's so quiet. Mine were always all or nothing.'

Sadie's mum has bleached blonde hair and smells like cigarettes. She gives me a brief, nervous smile and catches my eye, trying to work out what I'm thinking. I know this expression by now. She's trying to work out whether I have an idea about when the baby will arrive, like I have a midwifery crystal ball.

Sadie settles herself more comfortably and says 'Fucking

hell,' by way of a greeting. I laugh.

'Swear while you still can,' advises her mum. 'You don't want to be saying that when this little bubba's on the outside. What if that its first words?'

I grab her notes, 'Who's your midwife? Emma, I don't know her. She's written, "tough as nails" down here though.'

She's written nothing of the sort, of course, but it makes Sadie smile. After a few minutes, she rolls forward again and starts whimpering. I ask her if she wants some massage.

'Yeah, please...' I see her belly tighten and I press my hand firmly into her back and sweep it in circles. She moans, her voice lowering. I breathe in time with her. Everything seems to slow down and when she opens her eyes again she's calm.

I can feel tiredness threatening to take over and I'm crying out for sleep. I'm glad I'm not giving proper care, I don't think I'd be fit to. I excuse myself to make drinks and in the kitchen I gulp some more coffee, made fast and topped up with cold water, and hope that it doesn't make me shake.

We hardly see Emma the midwife apart from when she's listening to the fetal heart, as she's looking after the induction bay as well as Sadie. This suits all of us, though I am a bit worried in case I miss something. I don't really know what I'm doing yet. Then I remind myself that I'm just here as a birth partner, I'm not listening in to the baby or anything. I can't be judged on this.

Sadie gets bored of being on her front, so I set her up in the shower and find the projector in the cupboard, which fills the tiny bathroom with the same multicoloured, flickering stars that Jo and I used for Brenna. I hope Jo's here for a shift in the morning; I bet she'd choose to care for Sadie if she knew I was in here too and she'd be perfect.

I put the radio on and they're halfway through playing *Big Yellow Taxi*. In the humid warmth of the shower I can see Sadie start to disappear. During labour, something usually kept inside rises up to the surface, regardless of race, age or background. Women all have a different reaction to labour, but the expressions and noises come from the same cocktail of hormones. It's an ancient part of the brain.

Sadie is crooning quietly. It's a deep, not-quite-human sound. Or maybe it's the most human sound she could make. She braces her hands on the wall and sways her hips. I adjust the shower to make sure the stream is beating on her back. I think about the girl that I met in September and think how different her body has become. Her mind is different too. Sometimes you get a year in your life where everything changes and you grow up faster than you ever have before.

At 6.45am the sun starts to rise. I watch it through the open bathroom door as it fills the labour room and it's a particularly beautiful sky, orange and gold highlighting the peaks of the clouds. My fatigued brain can't help but take this as a sign that this birth will go well. I know this is just superstition, which is harder to resist because I'm knackered. But it's a nice feeling all the same.

I'm also hungry. I think I'll go and make tea and toast.

As I slip out I see Sadie has her face turned towards the corner of the bathroom and is in her own world, a wet, warm little cave, listening to *Take on Me* by A-ha. Nice one, Leicester Sound.

I go past the crowd of midwives who are gathering for handover and go into the kitchen. It's nice being here not on shift, free to do what I want. I put the plastic cups on the tray and the white bread into the toaster and stand warming gold foil packets of butter in my hands. I also find some sultana cake in plastic wrap; cake is always good in labour. That was one of Mum's rules. Jaffa cakes were basically a prescription.

Someone is standing at the entrance to the kitchen talking to one of the obstetricians. She's waiting for me to be finished with the drinks trolley, I think, so I hurry but manage to tip over one of the cups of tea. It goes everywhere. As I'm swearing and mopping it up she finishes her conversation, about turns and says 'Good morning, Chloe,' and with a jolt I realise it's Karen Hodgson.

She has no hint of tiredness about her even so early in the morning. She looks alert and efficient, in a white tunic dress, three silver nursing badges pinned to her collar. I feel haggard in comparison.

'And what are you doing here not in uniform?'

'Um. I'm a birth partner,' I say, off balance and still trying to soak up the spilt tea with paper towels.

'Oh right. Your sister or someone, is it?'

'Actually no, not my sister... do you remember Sadie?'

'Who? From where? What was her surname?' She wrinkles her nose.

'Williams.'

'Oh, you stayed in touch, did you? That's nice,' she gestures me into one corner so she can put her lunchbox into the fridge. 'I should be on transitional care but May called in sick. I'll probably ask to look after Sadie, seeing as I know her. That'll be nice, won't it?'

She smiles and my heart sinks. Her blonde hair is thick, wiry almost, and her makeup is perfect.

'Have you done many labour ward placements?' she asks.

'Just one. But I'm here as a birth partner with Sadie. Not in a student role today.'

'Do you know how many centimetres she is?'

'No. But she was six centimetres when she came in...'

'Right. And when was the last time she had an examination?'

'Um, not sure...'

She glances out of the door at the board.

'Four am. So she'll be due for one now. Perfect, I'll do it when I take over.'

Sadie is now out of the shower and wrapped in a towel, lying on the bed with her legs apart and a sheet over her. Her mother is holding her hand and I'm hovering.

'Will this hurt more than the last time I was examined?' she asks, looking at me while Karen sweeps her hands across her bump, feeling for the position of her baby. I've been trying to hint that she could ask for a different midwife, but she's not listening, whether out of fear or resignation I don't know. Maybe she's simply too tired.

Karen says, 'It shouldn't hurt much. Not as much as labour. You can tell me to stop at any time. D'you want to breathe some gas while we do it?'

Sadie nods and I set up the tubing for gas and air and coach her through using it. The rattling noise of the dispenser mixes in with the sound of her baby's heart rate as Karen listens in. It's higher than it has been, racing along like a train over rails.

'D'you know what you're having? Pink or blue?' asks Karen.

Sadie turns her face into the bed. When she can speak after her contraction she says, 'Don't know. Chloe said it's nice to have a surprise.'

I don't meet Karen's eye, but I can tell she's irritated by

this. She starts the examination and Sadie's moans turn higher pitched and she looks at me, panicking. I hold her hand. I suddenly have no idea what to do.

'You're still six,' announces Karen, grimly. 'I thought you were having too much fun.'

My heart is racing and I think *shit, this is my fault* and then I wonder what else I could have done.

'Shall I break your waters?' says Karen, 'Which should speed things up?' There's a hint of triumph in her expression and tone of voice.

Sadie is looking at me like I have all the answers. She starts crying. I feel horrific and say, 'It's your choice, Sadie.'

'Will it hurt?'

'There are no nerves in the amniotic sac,' Karen says, 'So that won't hurt, it'll just be like an examination. Maybe a slightly longer examination.'

She goes on, 'I think this baby might be back to back. Sat on your spine, you know? Can be a bit more painful, but I'm sure you'll turn it around. Now you've got the gas it should be fine.'

She rubs Sadie's shoulder.

'Don't worry sweetie. It'll all be okay.' Karen looks at me with the steely overhead light behind her and I gulp.

'Shall I pop your waters for you, then?'

Sadie looks at me, looks at her mum and then nods. Karen asks me to get an amnihook, which is like a long plastic yellow knitting needle with a sharp point on the end. I peel back the packaging, not touching anything so it's still sterile, and Karen takes it from me and immediately starts moving her fingers around inside Sadie. Sadie starts to scream. I close my eyes. I'm helpless.

No, I'm not.

I open my eyes again, squeeze Sadie's hand and say to Karen, 'Can you slow down please?'

Karen is startled and stops her examination. I walk over to the sink and run a washcloth under the cool tap and wring it out. I put it on Sadie's forehead. Then I tell her to look at me. She does and I breathe with her, in and out, in and out. I can feel annoyance coming off Karen in waves, but I don't care.

'Tell Karen when she can keep going.'

After a breath of gas, her shoulders and chest rising above her beautiful globed abdomen, Sadie nods.

Karen's fingers disappear again and Sadie tenses and grabs onto her mother's hands this time, instead of mine. Then there's a gush of straw-coloured fluid that smells of sweat and a lot like bleach, and it floods over the inco sheet, the bed sheets and straight off the bed.

Karen gasps as it's gone all over her, splashing down her apron and I think probably into her shoes, and I have to laugh. But I put my hand up to my mouth and stop quickly, because I know we're in trouble here. Karen is laughing too, but it's forced and only to save her from looking foolish. Under the laughter is irritation.

I'm standing in the shower with Sadie. I'm getting sprayed a bit, but I don't care. Sadie's mum is in the labour room with her head in her hands. I think she's sleeping so I've turned the main light off again.

I'm so tired that I'm beginning not to care about anything. All I want to do is lie down. I press my hand into Sadie's back where she wants to be touched, over and over again.

It's getting busy. Karen is also looking after a woman being induced. She comes back in. She's changed into some blue scrubs and has pinned all of her badges onto the V-neck collar. She looks at us both in the shower.

'Chloe, you're soaked. Go and get changed, please. Put some scrubs on.'

'I don't mind.'

'You're not much good to Sadie if you're tired and wet and cold, are you?'

I have a feeling of foreboding but I go out anyway, down to the staff changing room. I try and move quickly but I'm slow at peeling off the wet things. I leave them in a heap on a towel on the floor, I'll sort them out later.

I use a safety pin to hook through the V-neck to stop the scrubs top gaping. They don't fit that well.

Then I sit on the bench for a few moments, catching my pale face in the mirror. I close my eyes and sleep beckons and I follow for a little while and then I force myself to get up again.

When I go back into Sadie's room, everything has changed. Sadie is in a hospital gown and Dr Roshni is in the room saying, 'If you want something, you only have to say.'

Sadie's mum is nodding and looking serious. The radio has been turned off, the main light is on again and the window is open, letting in the sounds of a lorry turning.

Karen beckons me and I follow her outside. One of the healthcare assistants is mopping the corridor and she glances at us.

'Are you okay now? Clean and dry?' I nod and she looks me in the eye. 'We were just chatting about some form of pain relief for Sadie. The poor girl's struggling.'

I gulp and say 'Um, okay. But have you looked at her birth plan? She doesn't want anything?'

'Yeah, but that was before we knew she was labouring with a posterior baby. I mean, really. She's only sixteen.'

'But she talked this kind of situation through with me when she wrote her birth plan, so shouldn't we ask her about that?'

I always seem to be be a step away from war with Karen. As her voice is getting louder and more confident, mine is getting higher pitched and out of control. She's staring at me with one eyebrow raised.

'You've got an agenda, Chloe.'

My mouth opens and closes.

'Don't show yourself up, now. Let her make her own decisions. She'd do well to have an epidural. Women can end up with post-traumatic stress if you leave them in that much pain for too long. Have you thought about that? She'll want to look back on this day and know she was in good hands...'

I want to tell Karen that *she's* the one trying to make decisions for Sadie and if she knew her properly, knew how ballsy she is, she'd never dare. Instead I just stand there.

Karen looks at me expectantly. 'Have you got something else to add? Spit it out. We need to make progress.'

I don't say anything. She opens the door to the labour room and I think for a second I must have misheard, that she couldn't be that rude or that cruel, but she says, 'She's not your project, you know.'

The door bangs closed. I take a big breath and then look up at the foam-tiled ceiling, willing myself not to cry. The tiredness is actually helping with this. It's awful, but if I lean into the exhaustion I'm too numb for tears. I see a flash of the healthcare assistant looking at me with sympathy, but when I look around again she's taken her bucket and mop back into the sluice and I'm left in the corridor on my own, trying to summon the courage I need to go back into the labour room.

* * *

At 11am, Sadie is on her hands and knees on the mat, in a hospital gown with a sheet covering her lower half. She's declined everything pain-relief wise, not explaining why, with a flat expression and no hint of rapport, to the annoyance of Karen and Dr Roshni. I think she's scared of needles. Either that, or she really believed me when I told her about endorphins, the natural painkillers, and she wants to stick with her birth plan.

The cake seems to have perked her up a bit. Her contractions are more frequent, more like Brenna's contractions, long and hard. Karen is sat in the corner with a face like a dissatisfied gargoyle, doing her notes.

'You look like you're in casualty,' says Sadie, peering up at me.

'The scrubs? I know right, my colour.'

'Mum's asleep. She's snoring.'

'We'll leave her.' I'm jealous of Sadie's mum relaxing in her chair, but I think she realises I'm doing a good job of looking after her daughter and she's here for the main event. Maybe it would be more complicated if she was involved as well as me and Karen.

To me, Sadie looks like she might just be pushing. She keeps tipping her head down and closing her throat and tensing.

I concentrate on pressing my palm into her back. And I think she pushes over the whole next contraction, with little under her breath grunts, in a dreamy different space. I'm so proud of her. I don't want Karen to know. As I listen to the tea trolley rattling along the corridor outside I know there's something important about leaving Sadie be and not letting Karen in on the secret.

I wonder whether the bit of Sadie's brain that's in charge of her labour has it all planned out. Maybe it knows she needs to hide in this hospital, hide from Karen. I wish Mum was here. Sadie could do all this without worrying.

'You don't want the gas, Sadie?' asks Karen, briskly. This is the third time she's asked in the last hour.

'Doesn't help...'

Sadie groans and puts her head down and pushes again. It's totally silent this time, but I'm sure.

'Okay then sweetie,' says Karen, 'Time for another listen in.'

The heart races along and I count, *141, 142, 143* – it's faster than it was at the beginning of the labour. I want to ask about whether this is okay, but I don't want to speak to Karen. Sadie is lit up by the sun coming through the window and looks like she has a halo. I smile.

'You're so chilled out. You look lovely in the sunshine.'

'Mmm... Stay with me.'

'I will. Hang on, just let me look after your mum.' She's asleep, her head resting on the wall; she's probably been up for over 24 hours if she was supporting Sadie from the first twinge. I put a blanket over her and come back to Sadie on the mat.

After forty minutes I can smell fresh shit and Sadie is so far into the second stage that I bet we could see the head. It's crazy that Karen has missed all this. Every listen in has been between contractions and the baby's heart rate sounds fine. Karen has been busy and distracted. I think she's decided Sadie won't progress so she's not seeing any of the signs.

At ten past twelve, she comes back in, 'Right, sorry about

that, in with the inductions. Time for another examination. Can you get on the bed?'

Sadie is slouched over the birth ball, her eyes closed and her expression not registering that Karen's said anything.

Karen sniffs and says, 'Oh...'

She lifts the sheet and her eyes go wide. Sadie's perineum has flattened, and there's a small circle of dark hair visible as well as some red mucus.

'Sadie, your baby's just sat here!'

'No way! Amazing!' I say, my voice sounding fake even to me and I smile the most innocent, reassuring smile I can.

'Sadie, well done you!' I rock back on my heels and then help Sadie move, as she now wants to be on her back. I make sure there are pillows behind her, but I don't trust myself to look around at Karen.

Sadie's mum sits bolt upright in her chair, saying, 'What? Is something wrong?' and then Sadie holds eye contact with Karen, pushes and with the smallest of grunts her baby's head pops out with a gush of fluid.

'Oh. My!' Karen lunges forward and catches the head through the sheet, no time even for gloves, and the head turns towards Sadie's thigh and, like a magic trick, the entire baby slides out. Karen catches the baby with her bare hands and passes it through Sadie's legs and once Sadie is cuddling her baby to her chest, I cover them with a towel.

The baby is squalling, with a trembling bottom lip, outraged to be out in the light and cold and Sadie is saying 'Oh my God, you're perfect' over and over and her mum is crying over us. I'm smiling and laughing, hovering with a second warmed towel.

'Right. Birth at twelve thirteen...' Karen says, 'Sadie, did you want the injection in your leg? For the placenta?'

'No, she doesn't,' I say and Karen shakes her head at me.

'You had quite a prolonged labour early on, it might be better to, it'll help you stop bleeding. It could save your life and you're a mother now.'

Sadie glances up at her. 'I hate needles. Can we just leave it?' Karen nods and then catches my eye and gestures towards the cord clamp. I can see she has her hands covered in vernix so I start to open it for her.

'Why didn't you tell me she was pushing?' she snaps at me, under her breath, opening up the bowl set. 'You've made me look like an idiot.'

I don't answer. I don't even look at her.

The baby is huge, with his cord thick and winding. He's a he. I lean in towards Sadie and say, 'Do you know what you've got?'

Sadie looks between his legs and then looks at me and says, 'Riley. I've got a Riley.'

I lean over and look him in the eye. 'Riley.' He stops crying, just for an instant and then starts up again even louder.

Sadie has no idea that some babies can be a pain to feed; she just turns Riley's head and supports his neck. It all looks a bit awkward, but I think she'll figure it out and he's gulping. I turn the lights down and tidy the room, emptying the laundry bags and scrubbing down the trolley and bowl set.

I'm beyond tired. I'm floating. I think about how quiet Sadie was in labour, alarmingly so, and I think I've realised something about her. All of this defensive stuff, it's just an act. Underneath Sadie is quiet and introverted and thoughtful. I wonder if she's noticed this about herself during her pregnancy. She's going to be a wonderful mum.

When I've tidied everything in the room away I pull up

SADIE'S BIRTH • 157

a chair next to the bed and sink into it, watching Riley's full cheeks undulate, his hands opening and closing as he sucks.

'I'm sorry.'

'What?' She's focused on her baby, playing with his hair, his back, his little bum, immersed. 'Oh, don't worry, it's so weird how you forget about the pain as soon as it's gone.'

'No,' I say, 'About Karen.' It's warm on labour ward. I'm too hot and sweating, even in scrubs, and my hair is glued to the back of my neck.

'What about her?'

I think about telling her that Karen is a midwife because she wants power. She wants to feel in charge of women, a ward and the births. She's a good person, at heart, but she's dangerous because she wants to hand out medicalised care because it makes her feel important. And she wants me to fall into line. It's the wrong care and the wrong attitude. God.

Riley finishes and his head falls onto Sadie's chest, his eyes closed, drunk on colostrum. Sadie looks at me with her eyes shining in the dark.

'Do you want me to put him in his cot?' I ask.

'No,' she says, 'I'll hold him. Go home Chloe, you're well tired. Are they going to take me to the postnatal ward?'

'Yeah, that's right. You can go home whenever you want though, as long as everything is okay.'

I embrace her and Riley and kiss her cheek. I'm irritated I can't stay. I want to crawl into bed beside them and make sure nothing bad ever happens to them.

'You were amazing,' she says, 'I couldn't have done it without you.'

'Yeah, you definitely could have,' I say.

She smiles at me, shaking her head. I make sure she's got her mobile topped up and then go to leave.

I open the door and go and collect my wet clothes in a carrier bag. I put new clean scrubs on to drive to Dad's, which is not allowed but I can sneak them back in. Right now I'm so far beyond caring about the rules.

As I pass the sluice door someone pushes it open and I can hear Karen in there loudly complaining about me not telling her that Sadie was progressing. I can't hear anyone else responding. I keep my expression neutral and let myself out of the labour ward into the afternoon, and the cool air is wonderful on my overheated skin.

There will be consequences. Later, I will be afraid of what Karen can do and say. But right now I don't care. I can feel the fresh air in my lungs and know this is Riley's first day on earth breathing and I wonder if it feels strange to him, the transition between the powerful supply of his mother's blood, and his own breath, the filling and emptying of his lungs, the rise and fall of his chest.

I drive back to Lincoln Street, splitting puddles which are reflecting the sun. I'm not even afraid of falling asleep. Everything is spaced out, but my body is full of euphoria.

I imagine all the things that have led to this moment streaming out behind the car like a banner. America with Mum, being taken to talks with her midwife friends, reading birth books, talking to women. Her stroke. Dad's neediness. Starting to train here in Leicester. Sadie. It's never easy, but this is a shining, golden moment and no one can take it from me.

11

Calculations

Wednesday, 16th May 2001

I'm at Christopher's kitchen table working on an essay on 'Optimal birth environment'. It's a day off placement and it's a nice morning out there, but this needs starting. The deadline is in two weeks. I wasn't in the mood to begin with, but now I'm enjoying it. There's a load of good evidence for having a baby at home. It's a basic concept; of course mammals benefit from their own stuff and smells around them while they're having a baby. It's what I'd choose.

I don't even have a spark of longing for a baby at this point, but I can't help putting myself in the women's position. I imagine giving birth at home, in the lounge, the same room where Mum gave birth to Ali and me. I love the little flashes of insight you get when writing this kind of thing.

I'm drafting my conclusion, which is what I always do first with essays, when the doorbell goes. I ignore it as Narborough Road has lots of Good Samaritans and TV subscription people and other cold callers who go up and down, and I assume it's one of them. But it goes again and there's a knock too and I hear someone call, I think through the letterbox, 'Hello there? Christopher?'

I go to answer it, cautiously. I haven't met any of Christopher's friends barring one best mate he has from swimming who we've gone for a beer with. He'd clearly been briefed to be nice to me.

When I open the door an enormous man with squinting eyes and grey stubble is on the doorstep. He has a Leicester Uni ID balanced on a beer belly under a white shirt and he's carrying a lot of weight in his face. Even his ankles, in black socks and visible above brown leather shoes, curve outwards, showing his obesity.

'Hello. Can I help?'

'Yes, is Christopher in?' He smiles. He's very well spoken.

I realise that I have no idea if Christopher has told anyone at uni about me. I've been here for a few months and we've been together for well over a year, so I assumed we must have been seen out and about by some of his colleagues by now, but perhaps not.

'He's not in, I'm afraid. Are you wanting to leave that for him?' I gesture at the folder he's holding.

'Yes, alright. I'm one of the professors at the University. I came with something he needs, couldn't find him anywhere on campus. He does like to disappear! Are you a friend staying?'

'Something like that.'

'Oh.' he stops rocking and peers at me, looking me up and down.

'Well, I'll let him know you came.'

'Yes. I'm Dr Campbell,' he says. He holds his hand out and I shake it, feeling his clammy palm.

'Chloe,' I say. He stands looking at me for a few moments and it's a bit odd, so I say 'Well, I must get on with my essay...'

'Oh, are you a student too?'

'A student midwife.'

'Right. Very good!' He beams at me, pleased to have worked this out, and seemingly wanting to offer encouragement.

'Um. Thanks. Well, have a good day then.' I shut the door, relieved to see him go.

When Christopher gets back he seems tired and distracted, and after kissing me on the cheek gets on with making dinner. It's stir-fry and I do a few more sentences on power dynamics between professionals and women as the onions start to hiss. But my heart isn't in it and I decide I'm done for the day and come and sit at the breakfast bar and ask if he needs a hand.

'No,' he says shortly. 'It's nearly ready. Five minutes or so. You can get sorted for tomorrow or something.'

I can smell the fresh ginger that he's cut into long thin strips and added to the vegetables. We're having tofu, not something I'd ever really eaten in pre-Christopher days, but it's nice enough if you drown it in soy sauce.

'Okay. Christopher, did you see that folder?'

'What folder?'

He turns around with the rubber spatula in his hand and sees it on the coffee table.

'Oh.' He puts everything down and turns the heat off, wiping his hand on the tea towel.

'Dr Campbell came round, is that his name? He's a really big guy? He dropped it off. Who is he?'

'My PhD supervisor. He's got no boundaries or social skills, I'm afraid. Brilliant academic but horrible to work with.'

'Yeah, I sort of picked up on that.'

'What did he say?'

'Just that you needed the work and he couldn't find you.'

'He's not supposed to come around here unannounced. I

thought he'd stopped doing that.' He pulls out a thick wodge of papers. 'Oh, and he's rubbished a lot here that he told me to write, wonderful...'

'Can I help?'

'No. Chloe, what did you say to him? Did he ask who you were?'

'I told him my name, but I didn't say you were my boyfriend or anything.' He nods, reassured. I sigh. I don't want to upset him by pushing the conversation, but we can't go on like this forever.

'Do you not want them finding out?' I ask.

He doesn't answer, just goes back to cooking. He doesn't say anything else until he's put the meal on to plates and we're eating.

Then he says, 'They just don't know you,' as if continuing on from something I said a few seconds ago.

I'm not really sure how to respond to this, but he continues before I can say anything anyway.

'It's not like I go for eighteen-year-olds, like it was a plan.'

'Um, thanks.'

'Chloe,' he looks at me with desperation, 'People judge you for your private life. You know this.'

'Do I? Have you told anyone?'

'Well, not in so many words. It's none of their business.'

'I think it's really obvious there's nothing weird between us. You can tell when a relationship is wrong.'

'I'm not sure everyone at the uni sees it that way.'

He looks so miserable that I want to reassure him. But he might be right, I have no idea how his colleagues would react to us.

'My lot are different I think,' I say, considering. 'They make jokes but they don't really care. I think they're too young to take it seriously, apart from Jos.'

Poor Jos. I should phone her. She keeps getting bumped to the bottom of my priorities.

'It's hard enough in that office sometimes without giving them ammunition. I don't know, if we were married or something it'd be fine...'

I freeze and look down at the table. He's twirling a noodle around his fork, apparently oblivious to my discomfort. A sesame seed has got stuck in my throat and I take a sip of water and cough and the ginger makes it burn going down.

'Where were you today when your supervisor couldn't find you?' I ask, thinking he'll tell me about swimming.

'Oh, just across to the hospital. I had a patient I needed to follow up with,' he says, and then turns the TV on with the remote over my shoulder. It's a rerun of *The Office*, which I kind of hate. Ricky Gervais makes me cringe. But after a while I move my chair around the breakfast bar like Christopher and we watch it together. We don't really talk as we clear up, either.

Later on when we're in bed we lie curled around each other and I say, 'Christopher. You'd tell me if you were unhappy with having me here, right?'

'I am happy, that was never the question. Quite the reverse.' he says.

There's another silence. Then: 'If there's anything not right in our relationship, it's my fault, not yours.'

He doesn't hurt me but he undoes my dressing gown without even kissing me. I'm into it but it's rougher than usual and though he lasts a long time, it's far about what he needs. As soon as it's over he presses his face into my neck as we spoon and squeezes me tightly. Then he whispers 'I think we should have my parents around,' and I'm surprised. I had no idea what he was thinking.

I suddenly understand that today he was a little bit scared of losing me and I feel almost maternal, like he's younger than me.

'Ok,' I whisper, and I hear his breathing even out and know he's asleep. It takes me longer to drop off. I'm not sure what my problem is, but it feels off. Being this needed by Christopher is a combination of heady, powerful, and very, very worrying.

Tuesday, 29th May 2001

Today we're learning how to do drug calculations. We have an exam in a few weeks and we'll need to get 100% right to pass. One of the nursing staff is taking us for this lecture and she's good. She realises most of the class are het up about it so we're taking it slowly. The sums themselves aren't complicated, it's just that there's so much responsibility and pressure involved that you can make mistakes second guessing yourself.

I'm daydreaming, staring at the backs of the students in front of me who are all taking notes on drip rates and milligrams and fiddling with their calculators. Noelia keeps making silly strained faces at me and I smile back and shake my head. She's doing fine.

I struggled a bit with the more complicated atomic calculation stuff in my Chemistry A-level, but I quite like the problem-solving of this kind of maths. Dad was always quizzing us on sums when we were little and his arithmetic is brilliant, which is the case for most carpenters I suppose. The class is soothing and low-key, exactly what I want and need.

Today we should get our next placement timetables and I'm looking forward to seeing where I am, whether it's somewhere I know through Mum. I'm hoping to be out in the sticks in Melton Mowbray, because of the birth centre there.

In the coffee break I pour my tea, black because the milk leaves a sour smell on plastic and I've borrowed the thermos from Christopher.

Noelia comes back to our desk with an almond croissant and a cappuccino and we chat about her family back in Spain, who she's going to see over the summer. The lecturer starts handing round our timetables.

'I'll be swimming in the sea, early morning and late at night, otherwise I'll burn. Not used to it anymore,' says Noelia. Her voice is gleeful.

'Where d'your family live?'

'A little village on the south coast On a clear day, you can see Africa over the Med. I'll be swimming in the sea every day.'

'Try swimming in the sea here! My Mum used to take us to Norfolk.'

'Spanish people don't swim in the North Sea.'

'Yeah... Mum used to make us though. I can remember shivering on the back seat for hours on the way home.'

'Teo's staying,' Noelia says lightly. 'My family will be furious. It's the first time he's stayed behind for a summer trip. But he wants time with his friends.' The lecturer passes me my timetable from the stack and I thank her.

'Must be nice to have all that time off in the summer. Is he going to work somewhere?' And then I freeze. *Oh, no. Please no.*

'Are you alright?'

I shake my head, staring at the page. *Name of sign-off mentor.* 'Crap. Not good...'

'Chloe?'

'Yeah, I'm okay...'

'You look all freaked out.'

'Stay there, I need to sort something.'

I go out of the door and almost run towards the stairs, holding the timetable in a death grip. I know Rosie's in today, I saw her locking up her bike outside as we came in. This is not going to work; best I get it changed now, today. I hope.

As I approach the lecturers' office I can hear voices and without pausing or thinking I push the handle and burst in.

Rosie and Enid are sitting at their separate desks, deep in conversation. I hear something about *can't be involved* and then they both look up.

'Well, hello Chloe. I'm so glad we weren't talking about anything important,' says Enid. She snorts.

'Hi… I'm sorry. I didn't mean to…'

Enid turns away and starts to read something on her computer screen and Rosie looks at me, concerned.

'Are you okay? There's no emergency? You really should knock Chloe, we have confidential meetings in here.'

'Yes. No. Sorry,' I stammer, 'Really. I just… need to ask you something.'

'Ok. What's up?'

'Can I ask you privately?'

Rosie glances at Enid, who doesn't react. Then she pushes her chair back and stands. She's wearing a white lacy blouse that makes her look formal, in contrast to her dreads. She leads me down to the skills lab, opens the door and waves me in ahead of her.

There are four beds and a teaching dummy of a pregnant woman on top of one of them that I can see through the gap in the curtain. I breathe in. The hospital smell of drugs and antiseptic has somehow been imported into the skills lab along with the equipment. I wonder how I'm going to explain myself.

Rosie folds her arms.

'So what's up?'

'We just got the names of our community mentors,' I blurt out.

Rosie's expression is cautious.

'Right. Yes?'

'And I've got Karen Hodgson.'

'I see.'

'I... can I tell you this in confidence?'

'Yes. Unless I'm worried about the safety of you or someone else, it's always confidential.' Her tone is brisk.

'We just really didn't hit it off at that antenatal class, I think you know what I mean, d'you remember me saying? And then she ended up looking after Sadie in labour, who had a baby boy, a normal birth, by the way, but Karen just made the whole thing so difficult...'

I realise I'm rambling and criticising, not a good mix. Rosie raises one eyebrow and I stop.

I'm now very aware that I'm talking to a busy lecturer with lots of students to look after, not just me, and not just my year. I have no idea if Rosie has kids of her own, but I do know she's balancing research as well as lecturing. I'm about to sound like I'm asking for special treatment.

'Can we change our mentors?' I ask simply.

'I heard on the grapevine that Karen was asking for you specifically, Chloe. I'm really glad your friend had a good outcome. Karen's probably just impressed that you supported her so well.'

From what I've heard, Karen is furious.

The sunlight shines through the curtains and catches the blank, open eyes of the teaching dummy. I wonder whether Rosie has heard what Karen's been saying, whether she has some kind of plan.

'Karen just seemed to disagree with me about everything really,' I say, trying to summarise.

'Well, that's part of midwifery too. Working with people who see things differently. It could be great experience for you. You've done well on your assignments and placements so far, right?'

'Yes.'

'You're a good student, you have nothing to worry about. I think we'll use this as a learning opportunity for you. Karen's a very experienced mentor. You have her for four weeks, it's an interesting demographic of women over in Anstey and we're lacking mentors anyway. And she goes to Melton sometimes, the birth centre – you wanted that didn't you? Unless there's a very good reason, I don't think I can swap you.'

'So if there does turn out to be a good reason, I can swap mentors?' I ask desperately.

'We'd certainly have a meeting about it and treat it seriously, yes. But you're both hard workers. Maybe you'll be a good fit once you get to know each other better.'

Rosie turns towards the skills room door and I can see there will be no moving her on this. As she looks back at me, I feel trapped.

'Any problems and I'm here to listen though, okay? You should never feel like you're on your own.'

'Oh...Ok. Sure. Thanks.'

'Good. You're alright with this?'

I have to be, I think to myself in my head. But I say 'Yes, of course. Thanks for your advice. And I really am sorry about bursting in. It won't happen again.'

I follow her back down the corridor. Her shoulders are hunched and she looks thinner than last time I saw her. She waves me back towards the stairs and smiles to dismiss me.

I go back and apologise to the lecturer, as she's already restarted the session. After a bit more revision, we're given practice tests and the room is silent apart from the scratch of pencils and the tap of calculator buttons.

I start to work through the problems. Noelia mouths, *you okay?* at me and I nod back. She reaches out and squeezes my hand, wanting to help, unsure what's wrong.

I try and pull my brain back towards maths, to work out conversions and percentages. I force myself to slow down.

But I find myself staring out of the window, thinking, *really, I'm never supposed to feel like I'm on my own?*

Sunday, 17th June 2001

It's mid-afternoon and I'm driving home from a healthcare assistant shift, drumming my fingers on the steering wheel. The roads are quiet and it's raining, hard drops against the window. The countryside is beautiful with the crows, black soil and crops.

I'm doing shifts 'on the bank' now, which means I pick them up when and where they're available. They've had to replace me on Ward 15 because I can't commit to being reliable for my Sunday shifts any more, as placement will be starting again in a few weeks' time. I hardly make it to parentcraft classes these days either.

Christopher will be out late tonight because he's at a swimming competition and I can't face cooking dinner alone, I'm too exhausted. I didn't get a break at all today. I consider stopping at McDonalds and getting a burger and a Coke as a treat, but I'm not all that hungry and besides, the idea of eating Maccy Ds at the kitchen table after today is kind of depressing.

On a whim, I go around the roundabout and turn back towards Bradgate. I drive past a few brave families beginning to filter out of the country park in their wellies and anoraks, having spent the day walking with their dogs and kids.

As I pull up into Noelia's drive I see Teo is fiddling with an upside-down bike under the canopy of the garage door and my heart twists. I feel like this might have been a mistake. But Noelia has seen me from the top window and is already waving at me frantically. Teo grins at me as I get out of the car and am ushered inside out of the rain.

In the kitchen, the bitter rich smell of coffee is mixing with something savoury. My shyness disappears as I am reminded that Noelia extracts energy from conversation and loves having people over. She's perfect company for right now. She's in one of her hand-knitted jumpers, her bandana scarf wrapped around her hair.

'You like some *cocida*?'

'What's that?'

'It's supposed to be with chickpeas, sausage and chicken, but we do chickpeas and lots of veggies and herbs from the garden and things. Death-free cooking. You'll like it, you see.'

'Sure. Thanks.'

Noelia has a half-drunk glass cup of coffee on the table, the steel pot still on the stove, next to a saucepan.

She's been revising upstairs. I can tell because she's hastily dumped a few books and a pile of papers and scattered handwritten index cards on the kitchen table. I peer at them. They're about CTG interpretation. *Early decelerations with contractions, > 15 seconds, < 2 minutes...*

'You revising?'

'I have to. Us older-brained people have to keep going over things.'

'Oh, whatever. I revise all the time, nothing to do with age. It's hard, isn't it?'

She just smiles. She ladles *cocida* into one of her beautiful silver and blue bowls and passes it to me. The smell makes me realise I'm actually ravenous.

The stew is mellow and savoury with a hint of cinnamon and paprika. I eat in silence for a minute. It's wonderful. I'm about to compliment Noelia's cooking, but instead, as my mouth opens, I find myself asking 'What d'you think of midwifery so far?'

Noelia thinks for a second, unsurprised by the question.

'I wish we had more time with the women. England is very much better than Spain, but here, still, it's epidural, fluids, CTG for most women... very boring. Very disempowering.'

'Yes, I know. My friend I looked after, she nearly had an epidural pushed on her. And she did fine without it.'

'How did it go?'

I laugh a little.

'It was amazing. Sadie did brilliantly... she had enough and decided when to birth. The midwife who was on, however, I think she got angry with me.'

'Oh, honestly. Who could be angry with you, Chloe?'

'True. But she did.'

For a second I want to tell her everything, what Karen said and did to Sadie. How small she made me feel. How angry and scared I am about having her as my mentor. But I've never been the confess-all type and this is okay. Being friends with Noelia is so easy, I know I don't have to explain myself and make an effort. I smile and tell her dinner's wonderful.

'What have you been doing today? Working, that's for sure. You look tired.'

'Yeah, we did a resuscitation transfer over at Whitechapel, I was working over there as a healthcare assistant. The woman was in her eighties and you could see from the look on the faces of the nurses that they thought it was cruel to do chest compressions and maybe it was... I went with her in the ambulance.'

I falter. Noelia is looking at me with one eyebrow raised.

'The patient died.'

'All this, on top of training,' she says, 'I hope they pay you well?'

'The pay's okay. And they really need the staff,' I say.

'And what does your man say? Does he look after you?'

'Yeah. He does.'

'Can he cook?'

'Yeah. I do the cooking sometimes. But he's quite fussy about what he likes. He's out tonight. We're both really busy. He's got his PhD, I've got midwifery. I work a bit, he does his swimming training. It balances out.'

'Hmm.'

I'm going to say something about not having to pay rent and Christopher helping with revision, but the bead curtain bulges and Teo comes in, beads of water in his thick hair.

'Hey Chloe,' he says, and starts scrubbing at his hands.

Noelia tuts at the mess but he ignores her and says, 'How's placement? How's midwifery? You look tired.'

'Thanks. Is your bike broken?'

'Yeah, we're having an argument about returning gears. It's a black art.'

He smiles, then pours himself a cup of coffee and disappears up the stairs.

'Noelia, he's always so polite.' I say.

'You could tell him how it's going for you, Chloe. You're always so quiet. It's good for him to hear about work in the real world. He doesn't know he's been born sometimes.'

'I don't want to bore him,' I say, but she waves the thought away.

'Don't be silly. You tell him how it's going. All the gory details. He's not a typical Spanish boy. Back home in the village, we would never discuss birth with men, but Teo... we talk about birth, sex, anything. Spanish men are useless but I wanted him to be a feminist.'

'Well. I think English men can be pretty useless too.'

'Yes. English men don't talk about anything important, ever, believe me, I've tried. You can imagine what it was like for Teo growing up. He used to hate it sometimes. We were so different from all these English families, different from all the Spanish families, just ourselves. Ha ha!'

She laughs, more of a cackle really. I'm never sure how conversations with Noelia get so deep so quickly, but I'm glad of it. These days I think I'm more relaxed around here in her company than with anyone else. I'm getting sleepy, in fact.

'You're okay though, Chloe?'

'*Estoy bien.*'

'*Muy bien.*'

I have ten words of Spanish, but I love the language. One day I'll learn more. I rinse my bowl and leave it on the draining board and tell her I want to get going before the rush hour. I thank her.

'Any time. You're a good girl. Plenty of conversation and appetite.'

She kisses me on both cheeks and then squeezes me so hard I swear my eyes pop out a bit. And then I drive home, happy.

12

Barrier Method

I wake, suddenly, and I don't know where I am. For a horrible moment, I reach out into the void without knowing what I'll touch and then my eyes adjust and pick out the shadow of the spherical light shade and I realise I'm at Christopher's and I've been living here for six months.

I put one hand on his back and I can feel he's in a fetal position, having kicked the covers off. It's a warm night, too warm with both of us and the duvet, and as he gets up and opens the window I realise he must have been lying there awake.

Then he wraps himself around me. The breeze from the window cools me off and I instantly feel better though the traffic is noisy.

'Your heart's beating fast,' he whispers.

'Bad dream.'

'What about?'

'Can't remember... maybe it was the film.' We were watching a horrible horror flick before bed.

'You're not squeamish, though, surely?'

'It's not the blood. It's the screaming.'

'Which you don't come across at work?'

'Fair point, but it's not the same thing.'

'Why?'

'Believe it or not, they tend not to be as terrified as someone being chased with a chainsaw.'

'Oh.'

We lie in the dark for a bit. I sigh.

'I'm up in a few hours.'

'I can help you sleep...' As I relax into his touch, he buries his face in my hair and inhales.

I turn around in his arms and his eyes glitter in the dark. When he slides into me it's so intense that I whimper and he smiles at me like the Cheshire Cat and takes his time.

When he rolls off me, I settle into him again. Sleep is coming over me when he says, 'It's not the film. You're always tense before placement. You have bad dreams.'

'Do I?'

'Yeah, you don't always wake up.'

'Maybe you should wake me.'

'Yeah, maybe... how's it going Chloe? Placement? Uni?'

I think.

'This mentor on the placement starting tomorrow isn't my biggest fan.'

'Yeah? Why?'

I stiffen. There's no way I can tell him what happened with Sadie. There's a bit of me that thinks I should have been able to get on with Karen. I should have handled it all better. A real midwife would know how to turn her into an ally. But then he asks,

'Do you think it's harder for you? Is training different for you compared to your colleagues?'

I know what this question is about; we've danced dangerously near the subject before. He wants to ask whether it's harder for me because of Mum. I just shrug and hide my face in his collarbone, waiting for him to lose his nerve. He sighs.

'Can you tell me what happened yet? With your Dad?'

'Hmm. No.'

'Why? I won't tell anyone, you know that.'

'It's not that kind of secret. It's a stupid thing. It could be a dangerous thing. He's got to sort himself out. It took me ages to work it out, but I think this is for the best. He needs to sort his own problems.'

I'm trying to convince myself, but the guilt and shame rise in the dark like bile. I wonder whether Dad's awake, whether he's stoned, whether he's managing to feed Helga. And himself. I resolve to go and check on him as soon as I can.

'That's kind of the point of having a partner though, telling them things like this. I worry about you. What would your Mum say?'

I'm pretty sure Mum would have said Christopher should be supportive and not force me to talk about things I'm not ready to discuss.

'We never talk about your Dad anymore,' he says.

I change the subject.

'What about you? PhD stuff going okay?'

'Yeah, fine,' he shrugs, 'Just keep writing, that's all I do.'

I want to sleep now. It's only a few short hours before the sun will be up and I'll need to try and impress Karen.

'Good. You've found your thing, I've found mine,' I say.

'Midwifery's okay,' he replies, sleepily. 'For now. I think you can do anything you set your mind to. But it's not exactly good for quality of life or childcare if you want babies in future or anything is it? I want to look after you, Chloe.'

I hold my breath. We've never even discussed kids. I had no idea he wanted them. *I* don't know if I want them and I certainly don't right now.

I can't think how to answer. I lie in the dark listening to Christopher's quiet breathing for a long time until I'm sure by the rhythm that he's asleep. Then I get up and go to the bathroom to pee and wash myself. The moon is shining and a chink of light falls onto the floor, making a silver triangle on the tiles.

When I get into bed I can't get all this out of my mind and I'm afraid I'm going to be awake until I have to get up. I lie listening to Christopher's breathing, which occasionally turns into a gentle snore. I miss my own room, my own house. But this is home now. Christopher moves his head and stops snoring and eventually, I drift off.

13

Karen's Care

The alarm clock buzzes at me and I silence it quickly, not wanting to wake Christopher. He rolls over, putting his arm over his eyes to block out the light, and I scoop up my uniform and bag off the chair and go into the bathroom to get dressed. I look in the mirror. Once I've put some foundation and blusher on I look okay. I've had a grand total of about four hours sleep.

I close my eyes and sigh. Right. Come on then. I open my eyes and smile.

The Sure Start Centre in Anstey is off Papermill Road and my resolve to do anything I can to get Karen on my side, to try to learn as much as I can from her, is still with me as I'm locking my bike up. It's already warm and beautiful with a wide blue sky. I tell myself this is a good sign.

I'm waved into the building by an overweight, cheerful receptionist. Just inside there's a children's play mat with toys neatly packed away in coloured boxes. I walk past a busy main office and already the rows of desks are filling up with staff with headsets and black polo shirts and others in clinical uniforms in different colours.

I see 'Examination Room' on one door off the corridor and I assume this is where I'm supposed to go. I knock and I hear Karen say 'Come in!' and I push the door and wait for her to stop tapping away at the computer. It's not that welcoming in here; just a bed, a few chairs, magnolia walls and a scuffed poster teaching handwashing technique.

Karen gets up out of her swivel chair. She's a head taller than me and is in the navy uniform that I first saw her in at the parentcraft class. She oozes confidence. She looks like an NHS midwife off a leaflet.

'Oh yes, Chloe, you're starting today. How are you then?'

'Great!' I say, hating myself. 'Never better! Really happy to be here! Have you had your hair done Karen?'

I think she's had dark brown lowlights put into her blonde hair since the last time I saw her.

She doesn't answer directly, instead pointing to a coat hook on the back of the door, implying I should take my jacket off. I drop my backpack and as I'm struggling with my sleeves she says, 'Now Chloe, we perhaps didn't hit it off in quite the right way – but you should know I think you have the potential to be a good student midwife.'

There's a bit of me that wants to tell her where she can go.

'Oh. Thank you.'

'You will listen to me though, hmm? Take my lead? You've not been out on a Sure Start community placement before, have you, so you'll need to listen?'

'Um. No,' I say, hanging my coat up and making sure my fob watch is on straight. Then I look her in the eye and say, 'I know I've got a lot of learning to do and I'm looking forward to it.' I sound formal and fake, but she looks satisfied.

'And how long have we got together?'

'Um, four weeks? Exams are at the end of August and we finish just before then.'

'Just four weeks! Don't forget to get your sign-off book out then. I'm not one of these mentors who'll do it all on the last day for you,' she laughs, grimly. 'You can start by getting the clinic room set up, and then you could make us both a cup of tea. Just milk.'

'No problem.'

I take the plastic basket Karen passes me and I'm not really sure how she'll want things set up, but I know every item that's in there so I try to look busy and useful. I wipe down the couch and roll out a new layer of blue paper towel, set up the sphyg and put the sonicaid out as well. She continues whatever she was doing on the computer.

When I'm finished, I stand for a second, hoping she'll tell me what to do next. But she doesn't and I don't want to interrupt her, so I go out and ask the receptionist where the kitchen is and she points me through the main office to the break room.

'We all tend to have lunch in there too, duck,' she says and I thank her. Physios, nurses and health visitors all use this Sure Start as base camp. I'm glad about this as the break room should be full when we eat in there. I'll be able to escape from being one-to-one with Karen, at least for a bit.

When I've made the tea and am walking back with the mugs, there are a few pregnant ladies gathered on chairs outside the room. I smile at them and they smile back and one gets up to open the door for me.

Karen takes her mug without thanking me and leans back in her chair. Then she looks around the room.

'Put the dipsticks by the sink,' she says, pointing. 'You've done urinalysis before? Good. You can be in charge of calling the women in and doing that, then. Say the result out loud to me.' Her voice is brisk and efficient.

First in is Frances Brown. She's the lady who opened the door for me and she passes me her urine sample with an apologetic expression. It's light and clear and looks normal to me. I thank her and dip with a testing stick. These have little squares on that change colour in the presence of protein, which can mean pre-eclampsia or kidney damage; excess sugar, which can mean diabetes; and a few other things.

'It's NAD,' I tell Karen, as she's doing Frances's blood pressure. *No Abnormalities Detected.*

'Great.'

I wash my hands and hover as Karen does a palpation, unsure whether I'm allowed to ask to do one too. Frances's bump is small for a thirty-weeker. It looks to me like it's all hidden under her ribs. Karen doesn't say anything.

But then she starts to call things out, fundal height 29cm, baby transverse, not engaged but good fetal movements, and I write all this in the tiny grid that's within Frances's handheld pregnancy notes.

Karen finds the fetal heart with the sonicaid and the familiar beat fills the room. Frances smiles. I smile. I have an overpowering urge to ask about my pinard.

'Um, Karen, I have a pinard in my bag –'

'We'll do that later if there's time,' Karen says, looking over her shoulder at me, raising her eyebrows as if I don't quite realise how demanding I'm being, but she's being really nice about it anyway.

I feel like a bit of an idiot. I'm jumpy and nervous and I don't even have my normal start-of-placement excitement. I'm tired. But, oh well. I'm here. I'm learning to care for women with an experienced midwife and, in the end, that's all that counts.

14

Marston House

It's mid-afternoon and we're driving to the council flats, just north of Highfields, to do an antenatal check. I'm happy to be out in the community, but worried by the prospect of being trapped in the car with Karen all day. She's wearing me down. She keeps asking me questions about my life, what I like to do for fun and what Christopher thinks about midwifery, and I never know how to answer. It all seems very innocent, but each time I let something slip it comes up in conversation later as a dig. I'm nearly through this placement, just one week to go and I've been functioning like a machine, hating myself for being fake polite, palpating, auscultating and documenting. The main thing I am is mind-numbingly tired.

I still have twenty competencies to get Karen to sign off in my practice document. This is looming like a storm cloud. Without her signatures, I'll need to repeat the placement in the summer. If I don't get through that placement, I'll need to repeat the year and my suitability to become a qualified midwife will be called into question. If you fail two components, you're off the course.

This state of being has found its way into life with Christopher. I come home, tidy up, revise, go to bed early, set the alarm and creep out quietly in the morning. I think he's worried about me. I just want to keep focused until after this placement and my exams are over and then I can relax in the summer before I start on year two. I try to ignore the whisper that says Karen will never sign me off, at least not willingly.

Karen pulls up and parks outside the flats, broken bottles and wrappers littering the grass and garden beds. As we go up the steps a grim-faced teenage girl with cornrows and a buggy holds the door open for us and her toddler giggles. I smile back but they're already gone, down the concrete ramp.

The lifts are out of order, which makes Karen grumble, so I take her bag for her.

'This one's on a methadone programme. Her name's Sam. Keep your eyes open, it's dodgy round here.'

We trudge up six flights of stairs. Someone's pissed in the corner at some point judging by the smell, and there are cigarette butts and graffiti all the way up, but I've done a few antenatal checks at home now and I know how much better it can make things for the women to have a midwife pop round. Especially for those who feel like no one else cares, it's a wonderful thing to do.

We check the address and ring the bell and as we stand waiting I see someone has written *Sexy Sammi!!* inside a heart in black marker pen on the wall of the corridor. There's a bit of shouting that we can hear through the door and I look at Karen, who raises her eyebrows but doesn't look back at me.

Then the door of the flat is thrown open.

The woman who's answered is middle-aged, obese, with red cheeks and acne and black hair. She looks down at Karen's lanyard and ID, puts her hand up to her mouth and whimpers *'Please help'*. Then she disappears back into the flat. Karen follows her quickly and I shut the door behind us and walk in and see there's a younger hollow-eyed woman lying on the dirty grey sofa.

Karen starts to introduce herself, but she's cut off as the older woman says, 'Sam's back on the gear again,' and promptly bursts into noisy sobs.

'Shut the fuck up Mum...' Sam is painfully thin. She has the same black hair as her mother, though it's knotted and greasy, and she has a taut, pebble-like bump under a blue t-shirt.

Sam is slurring, and despite the fact she's lying with her feet up, she is grinding her teeth, tensed, ready to run. She looks at me with blurry eyes, like she can't be bothered with us. As she readjusts her position my heart starts to thud as I see there's blood on the cushion under her, spreading in a circular dark stain.

'Karen. Look.'

'What? Oh –' I think for a second she's going to swear, but she just crosses the room, drops down to her knees and says, all in one breath 'Morning-Samantha-are-you-bleeding-my-lovely?'

'Huh?'

She looks up at us.

'Samantha, you're bleeding – no, you're bleeding sweetheart, can you take your jeans off so I can see? Are you in pain?'

'No. Fuck off.'

'Shall I call an ambulance Karen?' I say and she nods and I start to root through her bag for her mobile. Sam's mum is still crying and while I'm looking I say to her, 'What was your name?'

'Me? Kim, What's goin' on? Why's she bleeding? I should have called someone, I'm sorry, I'm so sorry,' Kim is wringing her hands.

Karen sweeps Sam's t-shirt up and starts to feel around for the baby's position. I watch as the skin tightens and the shape of the baby disappears under taut muscle as Sam's uterus goes rigid.

'Samantha, you're contracting. When did this start? Have you got your notes? Do you know how much blood you've lost?'

Sam turns her face into the sofa and grunts, low and hard. Karen shakes her shoulder and then I think I hear her say *holy hell* under her breath.

'No, Samantha, you absolutely must not push. You hear me? Don't push. If your baby's born now it could die. This isn't even a qualified midwife with me, it's just a student, d'you understand? We can't rely on her care.'

I'm getting Karen's phone out of her bag but this makes me stop in my tracks. *Are you trying to scare the shit out of them, or just make me feel so useless that I can't help you?*

I look at Kim to check she's not panicking. Her glazed expression tells me she hasn't really taken in what Karen has said, but also that she'll be of no use to us. We're on our own.

I start to dial just as Karen says 'Chloe, call an ambulance. Now.'

The words make my breath catch in my throat and the phone is already ringing.

My brain has been hit with the urgency and I'm able to talk fast. I explain as quickly as I can and read the address and postcode from Karen's diary and the operator assures me a paramedic will be there ASAP, though I don't see how we're going get to Sam downstairs without the lift.

With tunnel vision, I see what must be Sam's antenatal notes sticking out of a shoulder bag on the other side of the room and run over. I open them up on the floor and start flicking through.

Karen is asking Sam if she's ever had a baby before and is fiddling with the sonicaid.

I find the information, my brain sucking it in and I hear myself say aloud in a voice much calmer than I feel, 'Gravida two, para one. One baby in care. Positive blood group. Child protection stickers. She's due in August.'

The other thing I see is 'history of depression and anorexia from early childhood'. *Oh, Sam.*

'When in August? Normal baby first time? Is there 'placenta praevia' or anything like that written on the scan page?'

I've heard of placenta praevia, it's where the placenta sits over the cervix, meaning a huge risk of bleeding and death during birth.

'No... can't see that. Premature birth last time, thirty-six weeks. Due 20th August now.'

'Right, this is a twenty-nine weeker,' says Karen, 'Put the notes down next to me.' I do so.

Karen is having a hard time, Sam is shaking her head and pushing Karen's hands away, but the fetal heart crackles out through the sonicaid and fills the room, quick and strong. Karen catches my eye and and my heart swells. The baby is alive.

'Mum, tell them to get the fuck off me!'

'Can you tell me what you took this morning Sam?'

'*Nothing.*'

'Did you take something extra because you were hurting? Has someone hit you, have you had an injury to the bump? Chloe, run as fast as you can, go and get my resus box just in case. While you're going, call labour ward and tell them we're coming in – can you hand over what's happening? Twenty-nine weeker, prem labour, drug abuse, bleeding. Got that?'

As I run down I catch the teenager again, shopping bags on her buggy, and I ask her to wait and hold the door and God bless her she does, wide-eyed as I rush past.

My heart is in my mouth and I fumble with the boot and put the resus box under my arm. I get through to labour ward as I'm running back up the steps. I tell them what's happening and the midwife on the phone takes all the details and then says *good luck* in a way that makes me scared.

When I get back into the flat Karen is putting a cannula in, which will be needed for any fluids and could be life-saving in terms of giving drugs later. Sam is trying to push her off, screeching at the needle. I go and stand next to her and try and talk soothingly.

'Sam, it's just a little scratch. This'll mean we can look after you and your baby much better –'

But she's having none of it.

'I don't wan' to go anywhere. Oh, whatever. For fuck's sake.'

'You are going in,' says Karen firmly. She hands me the four tubes of blood and says, 'Label.'

She's taken one for blood typing, in case a blood transfusion is needed, but I'm not 100% on the others. Iron count, probably, to check haemoglobin. Maybe a drug screen as well. As I finish writing out *Samantha Chelmsford, 20/10/1974* and the rest of the details on the bottles with shaking hands, I hear the ambulance pull up outside.

'Karen, how are we going to get her down? The lift's broken?'

She looks at me, 'Only one way down then, isn't there? Can

you walk, Samantha?'

'Yeah. Course I can walk. Can I have a smoke? Mum, tell them I need a fuckin' smoke.'

Karen looks appalled.

'I'll run down and meet the ambulance...' I say and grab Karen's bag.

'Ok. No, Samantha, don't have a smoke now, let's give your baby the best chance we can shall we?'

I leave her screaming about cigarettes.

The paramedic is in a green and white shirt, reassuring and broad-shouldered and he waves to me, his colleague still in the driving seat. I explain as briefly as I can.

'Well, shit,' he says calmly, opening the back doors, 'Has she got a line in?

'Yeah, Karen's taken bloods too... she's kicking off a bit. And there's no lift.'

'Try and avoid lifts anyway, to be honest. Nothing worse than being stuck in a lift with an emergency. Oh, here they come now.'

Sam is shuffling down the stairs screaming at Karen, who is steering her with a hand on her back, the resus kit under her other arm. Kim is behind them taking up most of the corridor.

'I want a smoke!'

'Looks more like she's had cocaine to me...' says the paramedic. He introduces himself to Sam, who's clearly not listening, and then asks Karen, 'Can we stop for a smoke? Do we have time?'

Karen looks at him with total disgust and says, 'I'd suggest we get going, *shall we?*'

'*He* said I could have a smoke, I'm going to go fucking mental without a *fuuucking* smoke...' says Sam.

'Sometimes it just makes everything much more simple in

the long run...' says the paramedic weakly, withering under Karen's gaze.

Sam tears her grip off Karen, leans against the ambulance, puts her head down and gives a long, guttural moan.

'Right! Is that a push? I see where you're coming from...,' he says, opening up the back doors of the ambulance.

Karen helps guide Sam onto the trolley and the paramedic is strapping her in. She doesn't look at me but she says, 'Stay here. We can't get all of us in. I'll come back or I'll send someone, leave the phone on.'

'Okay,' I say. The last thing we see and hear before the door closes is Sam curling onto her side and screaming at Karen that she's a fucking cunt. They drive out of the entrance slowly and then speed off with the lights flashing and we hear the siren start up as they pull onto the main road. The teenage girl is still at the door of the flat, staring, her toddler watching the ambulance pulling out while banging together brightly coloured plastic bricks in her buggy.

Kim has tears streaming down her face. I squeeze her shoulder, unsure what to say, and then jump like I've been electrocuted as a little red Ford screeches up alongside us.

Someone yells, 'Get in!'.

'Thanks, Kev!' Kim is still crying, but she wipes her hand across her nose and gets into the front seat 'You're coming too, yeah? Please come, we'll get you to the LRI.'

The man driving is wearing a grey baseball cap and a tracksuit.

'Karen's expecting me to stay.'

'Yeah, but we need you. Please, it's ten minutes away. She knows you, you can go and look after her. She's got such a kind face Kev, hasn't she got a kind face?'

Her eyes are pleading and Karen's going to need all the help she can get.

I can feel eyes on us; Marston House inhabitants are staring out of their windows. I get into the back and I've barely shut the door, let alone put my belt on, when the car accelerates like a rocket and I think maybe this is a mistake.

We shoot towards Humberstone Road, the wheels barely meeting the hot tarmac, past children in school uniforms and trees in full summer glory. 'No, slowly! Slow down! Kev!' I scream.

He ignores me. I can see his excitement in the rear-view mirror.

I close my eyes but it's still awful, my heart pounding in my ears. I open them again, clinging on to the seat in front of me, and he's weaving to one side, overtaking a bus, the expressions of other drivers furious and frightened.

'Kev, we'll get pulled over by the police!'

'Nah, it'll be okay!'

Kim has her hands over her face and is sobbing, 'She was such a good gel. No trouble from her when she was a kid. I keep trying to help but she just throws all it back in my face.'

'They might not let us in anyway, let's just get there slowly –'

'An' 'er first one in care and now this one… is she going to have the baby? Is that what's going to happen?'

'I don't know. We'll have to see.' I lean forward and put one arm on Kev's shoulder to try to get his attention, but I'm jerked backwards as we turn left past the shopping centre and I scream, 'Kev! *Slow down*. Do you know where the infirmary is? Just get us there. If you crash and we get hurt the midwives will be busy looking after us instead of Sam and her baby.'

This is not really true – we'd end up in A and E – but I'll try anything to get him to slow down.

'Okay. Yeah.' He reduces speed a little as we go past the community college, an older red brick and stone building near the centre. I catch my breath. 'It's safe though, I'm not going to crash. Once you've been a cabbie in Leicester, you know how to get out of trouble.'

We twist and turn through the city and, as he pulls up outside the infirmary, unbelievably the ambulance is just opening its doors. We've caught up. I'm shaking like a leaf.

For an instant, I feel the blood stop in my veins as I see the bulky figure of the paramedic with a tiny body stretched across one hand, an ambu bag in the other. He's pumping air into the baby's lungs, the paper thin skin covering the ribcage rising and falling. The baby looks pink at least. The paramedic runs in shouting at the receptionist to get the lift.

Kim howls. She sounds like a hurt dog and the few smokers on the pavement, who are watching the scene with alarm, look over at us.

I say. 'It's okay. We don't know what's going to happen, but the baby's alive. It's okay. They got here.'

'I'm going to go and help Karen. The best thing – no, listen to me – the *best* thing you could both do is go and park the car properly. Come up to the delivery suite. They might well ask you to wait. Stay very calm. I know I'm asking for the moon here, but we'll take care of her. We'll take care of both of them.'

As I scramble out of the car Sam is on a trolley being wheeled in and is shouting and trying to unclip herself.

Karen goggles at me.

'What are *you* doing here? Oh, *Christ*. Tell the family to stay downstairs. Hold the door please.' I do so.

'It's okay, they're parking the car –'

'Is my baby okay? I want to see her.' Sam is muttering, still struggling, and a midwife in blue comes out of the lift and starts clipping Sam back onto the trolley again, talking to her in a soothing voice, smoothing the pillow behind her.

Karen is giving the other midwife a lot of information very fast. I only catch a few words.

'We'll just get upstairs and have this placenta out. Had to catch the baby while we were still moving, there was nowhere to stop. And that resus, honestly, over one hand, I've never seen anything like it...'

My heart sinks. This information has hit Sam and she's beginning to cry.

I look her in the eye and put one hand on hers and say, 'Your baby looked pink. We just have to wait.'

Karen rolls her eyes at me and we get into the lift.

Afterwards

Karen is sat at the staff base desk doing the notes. I stand in front of her half timid, half furious.

'I'll go and tell the family what went on, shall I?' I say.

'Yes. Fine. They're probably in the Neonatal Unit.' She frowns and keeps writing. My head whirls. The words almost choke in my throat but I say, 'Can I get you a cup of tea?'

'Just milk,' she replies.

I turn towards the kitchen and she says, 'You're just so enthusiastic, aren't you?' I'm not sure whether I was supposed to hear or not.

A warm wave of shame starts in my belly and moves upwards and I flush. I breathe. Then I go into the kitchen, make the tea in a polystyrene cup and put it down next to

Karen on a napkin.

Without looking up she says, 'Tell me what you were thinking when you came here in their car.'

'I... they were upset and wanted me to come. They were coming anyway, I couldn't see much point just sitting there. I thought I could help maybe...'

Karen raises her eyebrows and keeps writing. I search desperately for other reasons.

'And... the experience would be useful and... isn't it better not to be hanging around St Matthews on my own?'

'When you're qualified that's part of the job. It's safe enough outside the flat – were you planning to only work in nice areas when you're a midwife?'

I breathe deeply. I look past Karen to the poster about breastfeeding on the wall and then I remember working alongside Jo. I try and imagine I'm talking to Jo and we've been on the postnatal ward supporting feeding, joking, up all night.

'No, I want to work everywhere.' I say.

'What if they'd have crashed? What if they'd taken you and my bag and tried to sell the ampoules in it? You put yourself in a very vulnerable position by getting into the car with two people you didn't know, in those kind of circumstances, relations of an addict mother, under an awful lot of stress.'

My cheeks burn and I hope she hasn't worked out how fast we got to the hospital, how dangerous Kev's driving was.

'Chloe, you're competent at times. You have a certain manner with the women, your skills and knowledge are coming on. But you take on too much. You don't know when to stop.'

A raw ache comes over me. I shut my mouth and try to look like I'm listening.

'You're a first-year and you're working under my PIN, d'you understand? I don't want to sound unkind, but it's my responsibility should anything happen to you or the women. And your friend's birth was mismanaged, if we're honest. I should have stepped in sooner and noticed she was in the second stage and pushing. Sheer chance that it was a good outcome. The one thing you can do is listen to your mentor and only take action if you are 100% sure whatever you're doing is in your sphere of competence.'

'Okay. Thanks. I'm sorry.'

She stares at me, eagle-like. I gulp.

'I'm sorry,' I say again.

'Good. Let's get on with the rest of today. We have one week left, yes? We'll look at your practice documents, what, Thursday? And if not, we'll make another plan and I'll talk to your personal tutor.'

I can't cope with this. I take a big breath. As I walk down the corridor some tears well up and I brush them away angrily. I can't be crying out here. But it's too much for my body; I can't shut down these feelings anymore and I slip into the toilets, sip some water by cupping my hands under the tap and breathe deeply, forcing myself back under control. I feel pretty nauseous, but I head back through labour ward, into the waiting area outside.

Kim is sitting on a plastic chair with her head in her hands. Kev is standing, leaning against the wall with his cap pulled over his face.

'Hi Kim,' I say, and she looks at me and sees my puffy eyes and expression.

'Sam's dead.' Her full-cheeked face goes blank and she says it like it's a fact, like the bottom has dropped out of her world and I feel horrific.

'No! No – sorry. It's okay. Everyone's okay. Sam's pretty out of it still, but she's in bed. You can come in and see her now. The baby is up in the Neonatal Unit and she's doing alright. I think they're sorting her out though, making sure all the bits she needs to breathe are there... best to leave the staff to it for a few hours.'

When we go into the labour room, Sam is relaxed and sleeping and looks much younger, her bird's nest of black hair spread over her pillow. She must have been a beautiful child with her fine features. I can now see her tiny freckles under each eye contrasting with her milk-white skin.

I squeeze Kim's shoulder and I leave her a tray of tea and a plastic-wrapped NHS sultana cake as she sits and stares at her daughter. It's not enough to bring her much comfort. But I think, *What else can I do for you? What else can I do for me?*

15

And Then

Twenty-four hours later, I'm back home to check on Dad. Finally. I've been meaning to do this for weeks and I can't put it off any longer. I leave my bag on the hall table and as I walk into the kitchen I'm worried because of the smell, but actually it's just a few plates in the sink. Everything else seems clean enough. Not scrubbed, but also not dirty. I rinse the plates and stack them in the dishwasher.

Helga curls around my legs and I pick her up and hug her to me. She purrs like she's got an engine in there and I'm reassured by the weight of her. She's still being overfed.

I inspect the fridge. There are actual burgers in there, not the microwave ones, as well as bread, tomatoes, posh cheese, milk and orange juice, along with lots of old takeaway containers. But that's every major food group accounted for.

'Well done Dad...' I murmur.

I put a load of kitchen towels into the washing machine for him and think I'll sit in my old room and drink tea and think and maybe revise for a while. I'm still exhausted, reeling, scared about what's going to happen on placement.

Surely Karen must be shaken as well after the events with Sam, however matter of fact she seemed? It doesn't get any easier, you just find coping mechanisms, is what Mum would have said. Maybe she's taking it out on me. I can't find a chink in Karen's armour showing any uncertainty or grief, though. In the car, after we'd left the hospital, Karen asked me what I wanted to do about my practice books again. *Sign them off,* I wanted to say. But I just shrugged and said 'I'll try my hardest.'

I think I might contact Rosie. She might understand. I've already stated my concerns; maybe there's another mentor I can work with. But I keep thinking about what I did in terms of getting into Kev's car and maybe I did screw up. Karen might be worried about getting into trouble; maybe getting into the car *was* a really stupid decision and any mentor would think so. It was a life and death emergency with a heroin addict, though, surely everyone just makes the best decisions they can in that sort of moment? I just have to hope Karen calms down.

I'm also thinking about the baby. The image of the pink body with black hair, draped across the arm of the paramedic while he forced air into her lungs from the bag and mask replays over and over, each time giving me a small spark of adrenaline. A limp baby is something that makes you shocked on a deep level. It's against the natural order of things.

Then the front door opens.

'Chloe? That you?'

Dad's come back. I wait for him to come into the kitchen and he creeps around the door like a wary animal.

'Hi. Shit! Dad, what the hell?'

He's got a black eye and I go up and inspect it and he stands there resignedly in his stained and misshapen polo shirt. The bruise is fresh, purple and swollen shut on the right and the skin has split and crusted above his eyebrow.

'Have you been fighting?' I ask.

'I got stung. By a bee. On my eye.'

'I wasn't born yesterday. When did you get beaten up?'

'It was a bee.'

'You're a massive idiot for getting into a fight and a bigger one for trying to tell me you haven't got hit in the face. It's really nasty, have you got something frozen you can put on it? Have you been to the doctor?'

'It doesn't need it.'

I open the freezer and rummage around. There are no peas, but I find a packet of chips that I wrap in a towel. As he takes it from me without meeting my eye, and sits down, I remember all the times he's looked after me. Walking Ali and I to school, bathtimes, dinner times. He's not a violent man, not one to get into a fight, which makes me even more worried about what he's mixed up in.

Before I left the hospital I pulled Sam's full notes, not the short handheld pregnancy ones, but the ones with her lifetime medical history. Despite all the trouble, I can't help but be glad my Dad is essentially a bit soft. Sam's had a lifetime of being terrified, starting as a baby, and the men in her life have been sexually abusive as well as physically violent.

Dad didn't even smack us when we were little and being naughty. When I was a teenager, he once told me about a time when he was at school and was 'given a good whacking' with a cane and then soaked with cold water in his sports kit and told to stand on a manhole cover outside. It was winter and he was barefoot. He was there for hours. This was a punishment for stealing a book about planes from the library. That kind of experience makes you go one of two ways.

He'd never get involved in telling off Ali and me, he'd leave that entirely to Mum. She'd smack us on occasion, if we really deserved it, but he never showed an iota of violence. He's trouble, but he's gentle. Not for the first time, I reflect that Mum loved him because he needed taking care of. She was good at being in charge.

'Is your eye anything to do with the stuff upstairs that I know nothing about?' I ask, abruptly.

'It was a –'

'If you tell me it was a bee again I'll give you another eye to match it. Why can't you just tell me the truth? Have you really got anything else to hide?'

He gingerly adjusts the chip packet on his eye and exhales with a little moan.

'Okay, so it wasn't a bee. I just didn't want you to worry.'

I snort.

He goes on, 'You remember Sven? He went a bit mental. We were stopping him from kicking off in the pub and he lashed out at me... it's fine, I'd much rather he did it to me than get in trouble with some pikey or the police.'

'Oh, so you're a punchbag for him. It's really not anything to do with anything in our attic?'

He just looks at me.

'If it was you wouldn't tell me.'

'It's fine. It's sorted.'

'Being a stoner... look, Dad, if you take a drug, any drug, that you don't need, every day, then it's not great. But more than that, it's stupid to put yourself at risk of gangs and the police and everything else.'

He says nothing.

'Can you not just stop? Just get rid of it all. They'll leave you alone if there's nothing here, right?'

'Chloe, I told you. No, really. It's not a problem and it's

certainly not your problem, so stop worrying, okay?'

'I don't believe you.'

'That's your choice.'

More silence. My heart sinks. I get up and look through the kitchen drawer where all the medications are.

'D'you want to take something for your eye? Paracetamol? Nurofen?'

'Nah.'

There's a nearly empty packet of co-codamol looking back at me, but I can't bring myself to ask him about it. I sit back down again and rub my eyes. I'm so tired.

'Are you working?'

'I teach classes at the college twice a week.'

'Right, good... are you having a drink? Tea?'

Reflexively, his eyes flick to the bottles on top of the fridge.

'Dad. Just have a cup of tea with me.'

He nods and goes through to the kitchen. I hear him fill the kettle. Helga jumps up on the table, next to the desiccated remains of a tiny table plant in a pot, well beyond saving. She presents her tummy to be stroked, her legs straight in the air with a haughty expression and I tickle her until she purrs.

I wait until Dad comes back and puts the mugs down.

'Mum would have hated you dealing.' I'm so exhausted that I don't care enough to be subtle. Maybe this is a good thing. He shrugs.

'How's Helga? She likes seeing you back.'

'She's getting fat, Dad.'

'She likes food.'

More silence. Then he smiles, tiredly, and I see the grey in his hair. He looks like he's smiling at me from a long distance away as he says, 'This bloke of yours sounds like a good catch.'

'Christopher? Yeah, he's a PhD student.'

He nods.

'Your type then. Clever. What's he researching?'

'Neuroscience.'

He gives a long, low whistle.

'And how's catching babies?'

I think for a second. I want to tell him what's going on, but I think it'll just worry him. And there's nothing he can do. Better to talk about something else, something nice.

'It's hard. Sometimes mind-blowing.'

He smiles. 'Yeah, You're like Mum. She lit up like a Christmas tree when she first started doing midwifery. She used to have breaks from it on holiday or when she was in college and she'd miss it and dream about it. She'd wake up saying things like 'You're doing really well,' or 'Can I listen in?''

I try and cling on to this thought, feeling a bit sick. I think I'm nauseous because I'm so tired and worried. As I finish my tea, Dad tells me old stories that I know well, of Mum being called away from birthday parties, getting up in the cinema in the middle of a film and people complaining and her shouting there was a baby coming, to mass panic. Once she pretended she had to go when she was at one of Ali's awful parents' evenings, leaving Dad to pick up the pieces. She seemed to have a lot of fun with it, as well as the struggles.

If I can get through this stretch with Karen, I'll be able to love it all again. It's good to have this reminder.

At the door, I hug Dad and he surprises me by tightening his arms around me, squeezing me in a bear hug and burying his face in my hair. He smells a bit musty but also of deodorant, with only a faint hint of herby, unsmoked weed.

'Come back soon, okay?' he says.

Before I left he told me that Ali's been hanging out with my old crowd, with Mia and Hamza, going to lots of gigs. He doesn't say anything about Jos though. I bet she's stopped going out to bars and nightclubs entirely. I feel guilty about not being in contact with Jos, except by text, for the longest time. But her messages seem pretty happy and I know that as soon as I make proper contact it will be like no time has passed at all. She's that kind of friend.

If only all problems could be solved as easily.

I couldn't bear to have the argument again so I didn't check the attic. It's obvious he's been beaten up. I don't want to call the police in case I pull the whole situation down on his head and maybe even on mine, but the anguish I feel over leaving him is awful.

But then my own concerns about placement and midwifery and Christopher come flooding back in and I remember I've washed my hands of him.

Sam's baby is cocooned in an incubator, an orogastric tube for feeding placed in her nose, secured with a small piece of tape. With her mask and crinkled tubing attached to the breathing machine, she looks like a tiny, unearthly fighter pilot in a cloud of blankets. Her rib cage is rising and falling and her almost transparent skin set with spindly blue veins reminds me of an autumn leaf. I've ridden over to the Royal on my bike and come straight to the neonatal unit and a nurse is hovering over my shoulder.

'Rough start,' she says.

'Yeah. I was there,' I reply.

'Oh really? Gran came up once but mum's already

disappeared from what we hear.' Her tone is disapproving.

'That's a shame. I was hoping to catch up with her,' I say lightly.

She grunts.

A machine starts beeping and she removes the sats probe, which measures blood oxygen, and replaces it on the baby's other foot. I can see she has no interest in Sam. Maybe that's a good thing. Maybe all her attention needs to be here.

'How's she doing?'

The baby stretches her arms wide and then pulls them back in again, shakily.

'See that? She's got a bit of a tremor going on, d'you see the jittering? We're keeping an eye. She'll be withdrawing at some point, it'll be about managing that. She'll withdraw from the different drugs at different times. Heartbreaking.'

'Yeah. It is. I'll pop in again if that's okay and see how she is?'

'I'm sure that's fine. What are you, first-year, second-year?'

'First year. What'll happen to her?'

'I'm not sure. Mum's an addict, is she? Sometimes they try to place the babies with family. Otherwise, we'll nurse her here until she can be fostered or adopted. I've not heard what the plan is so far.'

'She's so lovely...' I say, looking at her dark hair and tiny, perfect fingernails.

'She *is* a pretty baby isn't she?' The nurse looks proud, almost as if she's responsible for the baby's good looks. 'They're often like little old aliens at this stage, but she's a cute wee thing, aren't you?'

I thank her and head to the labour ward, just to make sure Sam really has gone. The coordinator tells me they barely persuaded her to stay for one night and in the end she wouldn't go to meet her daughter.

'She was still bleeding quite a bit really, terribly dangerous. I think her own mother is there with her at home though, what was her name?'

'Kim.'

'Good-o, I'm glad there's someone there for her. There was just no way that mum was staying.' She leans forward conspiratorially. 'She kept calling us all the c-word. As long as she doesn't have a haemorrhage though, she'll be fine obstetrically. Tottered out in heels, poor love. Bit of a lost soul. Poor thing.'

'It's not really her acting like that, though, is it? It's the drugs,' I say.

'Mmm.'

She's already tuned into the board again.

I go to the loo, pee, wash my hands and as I'm standing there thinking about Dad and his stupidity and the bleakness of some people's lives and whether it is their fault or not, I'm looking at the hefty pack of hospital sanitary pads which are left in the bathroom. They're free for us to use – one of the few NHS perks – but no one does apart from in emergencies, because they're like having a mattress in your underwear.

And then I turn my head and there's a long, terrible pause where I don't think about anything but the date. And, with growing fear, I think about how long it's been. I freeze. It's heartstopping. I feel like I'm choking and there's a ringing in my ears.

I'm staring at the blue teardrop on the packaging. I haven't bought any for... how long? *Wait,* I tell myself. *Count. You don't know.* But I do know. I'm really beginning to panic. My heart is pounding as I think about my calendar and the days jumble up into a small, confused pile in my head.

I look in the mirror and I look neat and professional, in my jumper and lanyard. I look like how I always hope to look on the labour ward, able to handle responsibility. Not like a student midwife who has just realised that through her own carelessness, she hasn't thought about her own period in months.

Christopher. What will Christopher do? Ali will laugh. Nanna will be so disappointed in me. My throat is tightening. My chest feels like it's been hit. Five, six weeks. Eight? *Ten?*

I watch myself like I'm outside the situation, floating above it, and I grope for the hand rail. The emergency buzzer goes off outside and I hear staff run, footfalls like a sudden hailstorm, to the other end of the ward. I don't want to be spotted by anyone; the healthcare assistants and a few of the midwives know me by now.

I walk back out of the changing room to the sluice. I watch the door, wait a few seconds and look around before pushing it open. It's empty. I'm flooded with despair. I can't just go into a pharmacy and get a pregnancy test, I could be seen.

But what am I doing here, stealing a test, when I'm already at risk of failing this placement? I can't think what else to do. I take a flimsy white and blue plastic strip out of the cupboard and put it in the pocket of my jeans.

Then the door opens and I jump violently, it's one of the healthcare assistants. She's busy, her head full of what's going on outside, so I don't think she saw my reaction. I try to smile.

'Chloe, are you here helping? Just we've got a lady going to caesar and we could use another pair of hands,' I'm about to follow her on autopilot, but she peers at me, at the same time as leaning over and scooping up some pads and the scales for weighing blood loss onto her trolley, 'Actually, never mind, you're upset aren't you?'

I nod, wordlessly, unsure what else to do.

'Is it Karen?'

I gape at her.

'No. How did you know...?'

'Oh, Karen's a pain to all her students. Don't worry about it love.'

She stands up and looks at me with a serious smile, 'Chloe. You need to talk to a midwife you trust.'

I don't say anything.

'Look... I'm in the middle of this theatre prep. But you can come and find me later, if you want, right? We can talk it though? I won't tell anyone, I promise.'

'No! I mean... thanks... look, that's really kind of you. But Karen's okay. Really. If I was in a right state and you were free I'd ask for your advice, definitely, but I'm okay...'

She pushes her trolley and I hold the door open for her.

I can see I've offended her a bit by refusing her help, but she's busy anyway, needing to get on. Before I know it she's pushed the trolley away and I shake my head and walk out of the labour ward without attracting any more attention.

Later, at Christopher's, it's quiet and I'm on my own, thank God. I don't think he'll be back until the evening. I sit for a long time in the lounge, trying to conjure images of any bleeding I might have had in the last few months, trying to will a missed period into existence. I know my tampons have been at the bottom of my underwear drawer for at least seven weeks and I haven't bought any pads for at least that long. Maybe I've been so stressed that I don't remember? It could have been a really light one, just a day or so. But I just don't think it happened. It's possible I've been so stressed my periods have stopped.

But it's also possible I missed a pill. With night shift jet lag, I can remember at least one time when I forgot and then took it late, but I might have miscalculated by a day, which should have still been safe, but it might have been 48 hours late instead of 24.

I think about Ali. I wonder if I should phone her. But I'm pretty sure she'd end up making me feel even worse, she's so blasé about anything like this. I bet she's been in this situation a few times. I stop myself and remember Ali has the implant, which she started using years ago. She's happy with it because she doesn't get periods at all.

I have the test in my hands. I know how these work; they're not the same as the big plastic clunky things you buy at pharmacies. They're cardboard strips covered in a thin film. If it's positive, there will be one blue line to show the test is working and one to show the presence of hCG, human chorionic gonadotropin.

Eventually I get up on unsteady legs and go into the bathroom. I'm shaking hard from the adrenaline, making it difficult to do up my belt, and as I pull my jeans back up I notice I've lost a bit of weight. My belt buckle is on the last notch. Surely if I was pregnant I'd be a bit bloated, maybe even gaining?

I close my eyes and take a big breath. When I open them again I look at the test on the sink.

The two blue lines are thick and heavy. Like an equals sign.

The reality of the situation spirals down on me and I sit on the floor.

It's unreal. I lived in an alternate universe for about two years after Mum died, knowing she was dead, but in a state of disbelief about how cruel life could be. Then I got to a certain level of acceptance and thought I was back on the right side of the tracks. And now I'm here. I'm numb and dizzy and unbelieving and there will be so many more emotions to come.

What would Mum say? She'd say it was my choice, she wouldn't be ashamed, and she'd be devastated that I didn't want to call my sister.

I shouldn't feel guilty. Maybe it's no big deal and in a few weeks I'll barely think about it. Ali would say that. Jos would talk about the Qu'ran.

Maybe I could steal something from the drugs cupboard at work and sort this out myself. I have a horrible protective, nauseous twinge at the thought, both because I could get caught and because it will involve losing something I've only just realised I've got. But this is a stupid, undo-able plan anyway, because you need so many bits of paper signing to get them.

I can't make any decisions today, even about how I feel. It's too fast.

As I lean against the bathroom wall and stare at a tiny speck of black mould on the shower curtain, I have the crushing realisation that Ali has dealt with adulthood far better than I have. Despite everything, she's handled the responsibility of sex and independence. She's tough and streetwise, and I'm not.

16

Case Review

I'm getting out of bed, trying not to wake Christopher. Karen will be picking me up on London Road today and we're going to a case review. I can see through the crack in the blinds that it's already a glorious hot blue day at 7am. Here in the bedroom it's cool and smells of warm skin.

I kiss Christopher on the cheek. I was in bed last night before he got home. He rolls over to doze for a while longer, as he always does if I'm getting up before him, but this time he opens one sleepy eye and smiles at me, before closing it again.

It occurs to me that we get on best in bed, when the lights are off or when we're half asleep, in any state that means our bodies are communicating more than our minds.

He's sleeping beautifully, one hand up over his face. I wonder what I should do. The traffic rattles past. I want to talk, I want to scream, I want Christopher to wake up and ask me what's wrong.

As I put my uniform on in the bathroom, I have to stop and concentrate and hold on to the sink to pull myself together. I don't know if this intense nausea, coupled with pain in my stomach, is shock or morning sickness. It's appeared since I realised.

I carefully apply foundation, dotting it around my eyes and rubbing it in. I think about when I started this course eleven months ago, how proud Nanna was to see me in my uniform, how hopeful I was that the hard years were behind me. I almost snort; never think that, it will come back at you if you think the hard part's over.

I try and imagine what Nanna's expression will be when I tell her I'm pregnant. Maybe it could work. Maybe I could even still be a midwife. I could take one year out and then rejoin the cohort below. It might get Karen off my back. I shudder as I imagine her satisfied, condescending smile at hearing the news. I remember what Christopher said in bed about childcare. He's older. He wants a family and he could get money and support from his Dad until he finished his PhD. He'd want this baby and who am I to make that decision for him? But I can't trust that he would still want me to be a midwife. And then there's the sense of wrongness I feel when I think about being with Christopher forever. Is it normal to be so scared of committing to someone? Maybe it's just a huge step and I wasn't expecting any of it. Maybe I'm in no right mind to think about this.

I wash my hands to make sure there's no trace of makeup on them that could be transferred to my uniform, before straightening my collar. Then I take my placement backpack and head out of the flat, over the road and start walking through the university and towards the station.

I know that as soon as this decision belongs to Christopher as well, it will terrify me.

I am beginning to realise that it might not be true that I don't need people to talk to. But I can't think of anyone I want to tell.

* * *

'Okay?' Karen has her hands on the steering wheel and is staring at me.

'Fine,' I mutter, 'How about you?

'I'm always fine.' As she pulls out into the heavy morning traffic, cab drivers edging in and out of the station and buses kicking out soot, I have a sense of not really being here. The smell of her perfume and the pollution from the busy road combine into something vile. I'm nearly heaving.

Karen says, 'So, a case review. Have you been to one before? D'you know what they are?'

'It's about child protection, right?'

'Well, yes, this time it is, but it's not always. This is for Sophie Brooks. Do you remember in clinic? She's an ex-drug addict? She used to have an abusive partner, he's in prison now.'

I can't concentrate or think of anything intelligent to ask, or even remember meeting this woman.

'Sophie's children were added to the register. This review is more about the possible neglect of her new baby than anything else, okay? There'll be social workers, her children's teachers, possibly a health visitor. Those kinds of people. We'll just have to see who turns up.'

The motion of the car isn't helping. I'm getting lightheaded.

'Oh, right.'

'Yes, it's very sad, isn't it...you have to feel for them.'

'Mmm.' I don't trust myself to look at her and keep my expression neutral so I stare straight ahead.

'Still, she might be all over the place, but she's trying not to be selfish. She's trying to give her kids and this poor new bubba a chance.'

Sweat prickles under my arms and I know I'm flushing.

Without meaning to, I meet Karen's eye in the car mirror and she's sorrowful, but underneath that there's triumph and I look away fast.

We drive in silence until we arrive at a small, beaten-up school in Beaumont Leys. We park near the pool and there's a swimming lesson in progress. You can smell the chlorine and hear the kids screeching and splashing behind the wooden fence.

For one second I am caught off guard in awe of this tiny, precious thing I'm carrying around inside me. If I leave it be, it'll turn into a child, like one of those behind the fence.

We make our way into the school and find the empty classroom where the review will take place. We're the first ones to arrive. A pretty receptionist brings us mugs of tea and I sip slowly and try to build my defences.

The room fills: a social worker, two teachers, Karen and me and the health visitor. The social worker sits at the head of the table.

'Thanks for coming all. I'll just sum up quickly if that's okay? I know we're all aware of Sophie's background, I think most of us have known her for a long time.' The social worker is in jeans and a checkered shirt and her hair is brushed but still damp from washing. 'Okay, so from our point of view Sophie has improved in great leaps and bounds. The teaching staff report the twins have better attendance than in any previous years and are here by 8.30am the vast majority of the time. There are no problems in the family with the hard drugs anymore.'

One of the teachers frowns and makes a note. The health visitor and the teachers give similar reports. The twins' teacher from year three says Sophie has even been doing their maths homework with them; the extra praise and correspondence each week has worked like magic.

Karen is asked for her point of view and she says, 'I can't report any issues with antenatal care. She's always on time, seems engaged in the pregnancy, she's still a smoker but otherwise makes appropriate choices... she says she's given up 'getting high off of weed' as she puts it.'

I look at the social worker and my heart drums in my ears at the mere mention of weed. Like a pebble on the beach, my emotions are changing position as each new fact washes over me. I have almost no control this morning and I see Karen raise her eyebrows at me. I must look tense and pale.

I flail around for a solid subject to think about, to ground me. Exam revision. A good thing to be thinking about, anyway. *Ferrous sulphate and fumarate,* I remember, *folic acid, syntometrine, vitamin K... right patient, right drug, check patient wristband, date of birth...*

I'm starting to get dizzy. I've never passed out before, but I can imagine what it might feel like now. I stare out at the sky and rub my forehead, willing the blood to my brain.

I mean to tune back into the conversation when the subject changes, but it's over faster than I realise and ends with, 'When this baby is born we'll call for another case review. When will that be, Karen?'

'Well, she's due in about eight weeks. So anytime from about halfway through September to halfway through October would be typical, but really, any time with her would be possible. She was early with her twins.'

There's a bit more talk about dates and times and then that's it, everyone starts to get their folders and pack up.

When we get back into the car, Karen drives in silence for a while, then says. 'You do look pale today.'

'Yeah. I think I'm just tired,' I respond.

'When do you have your practicals? Your OSCEs? On Friday?'

'Yes.'

'Are you going to be perky enough to do those? What are they on?'

'They could be on anything we've covered so far. Anatomy and physiology. Medicines management. Labour care.'

'Oh, of course – you're clever, aren't you, so you're confident. Well. Good luck. You'll probably have that bit sorted.'

She considers.

'You have some funny ideas. It's just whether we can get you through this placement or not. I hope so.'

I snap back to the present and look at her. *You hope so?* She's smiling at me like she can read my mind.

'Were you listening in there? You looked all over the place, staring out of the window. I thought you were going to faint at one point.'

I bluff, a hollow feeling rising in my throat. 'Yes. It's just a hard situation with Sophie, isn't it? Upsetting.'

'If you're on the job, you need to be listening, Chloe.'

We pull up on Appleby Drive, where sweetpeas are climbing trellises and sunflowers in pots are staked with canes. Two mothers are out for a lunchtime stroll pushing their buggies up the hill towards the cafe.

Karen sighs. 'It is upsetting, yes. You'd think a mum would do whatever it took to protect her baby, her own flesh and blood. But there we are. I'm sure Sophie's doing her best. And she's actually doing quite well at the moment.' She folds her hands in her lap. I have mine clutched together so hard it hurts. I can't think what to say.

'Your first year is all about learning the basics,' she goes on. 'If you're not well, or not coping, you should take time off. Your personal tutor can always add on an extra few weeks at the end of this placement during your summer holiday. And if you don't have time to get them in, or you don't pass, it's nothing personal, you can retake the year. Might be the making of you. And you know, if midwifery isn't for you, finding out sooner rather than later is for the best.'

Karen gets out of the car and starts rummaging in the boot to find the postnatal bag. I sit for a second, shaking.

I join her on the step and as we wait for the door to be opened by the elated first-time mum who we've come to see, I force my expression to be calm and positive and professional.

Thursday, 26th July 2001

Karen and I are on a long shift and should be out in the community, but we've been called into the labour ward to make up the numbers of staff. By 2pm the emergency buzzers are going off over and over, in different rooms, like whack-a-mole or a horrible parody of a quiz show. There's something serious going on in the critical care area; the adult resus team were here.

Our woman has an epidural and is sleeping the irritated half-sleep of someone connected to many drips and wires. Her husband is in the chair next to her and is blustering and unsure of me.

At one point he even reaches over and touches Karen's hand and says, 'The student won't be left alone, will she?' as if I can't hear. Karen smiles at him and says, 'Well, I may have to pop out for a second or so, but don't worry. She's not in charge of anyone's care yet, she's just a first-year.'

I stutter, drop things, and when I try to draw the little biro crosses that plot out the fetal heart on the chart, I can't follow it and I put in the wrong times. I cross it out so much that Karen rips up the page and asks me to start again.

'You're not with it today,' she says. 'Pay attention.'

The baby's heartbeat thunders on in the background until a contraction starts and then it slows and we all fret. Our attention must be on that. But I can't get my thoughts away from my own lack of ability to do a single thing right. My brain is full of fuzzy panic. I'm not letting myself think about anything other than this afternoon, but it's not helping.

Karen goes out of the room to get a new Y connector for the drip as it keeps blocking and alarming. She also needs a new pack of fentanyl and bupivacaine for the epidural infusion. The CTG machine starts beeping. The fetal heart is at 120 beats per minute and sounds like a trotting horse. I smile at the dad, though I'm sure it's more of a grimace, but he's concerned and asks me to go and get Karen. I silence the alarm.

'She'll be back in just a moment.'

'All the same. Now. Please. I'd rather you went and got her than set that buzzer off.' he says.

I'm not sure about leaving the room; the fetal heart could dip and there would be no one to call for help. But he's strident and I slink out feeling ridiculous.

'Um. Hi.'

The coordinator is standing at the white board, looking like she's considering a giant game of chess. She doesn't look round, just writes something into one of the boxes.

'D'you know where Karen is?'

'Sluice,' she says, without looking at me.

I walk down the corridor and as I go to push the sluice

door open I can hear Karen in there over the sound of running water.

'The point is, some of these young girls come in to be midwives and they lack life experience,' she's saying.

I freeze with the door opened just a crack and see her in there with another midwife, both of them leaning against the stainless-steel counter. My stomach clenches. 'Anyone can make mistakes, but some of them are just far too young. They don't know how to organise themselves or when to stop. It's not fair on them, actually, or the women. They're still working out who *they* are as people. And if they have too much going on in their lives to fully invest in their training... well, I'm blaming the admissions team, personally. Perhaps 25 years should be the youngest they go down to, though it does depend on the person, doesn't it..?'

'We used to have to do nursing first,' says the other midwife, 'Lots of scrubbing out of bed pans, that kind of thing.' She's older, still has a plastic apron on from her delivery room, and looks hot and irritated. 'It puts you in your place, gives you time to think about the role and if you want it that badly,' she goes on, 'Frankly, it's easier to train once you've got a few skills under your belt too. Knowing normality's all very well, but it's not the way care's going is it? All these women coming in with so many medical problems across their pregnancies.'

'My one's got all kinds of issues,' says Karen, 'For the lack of a better word, she's troubled. She's never said it but you can add it up. You can see it on her face. She's got family issues, a recent bereavement of a parent. It's just not fair to her and it makes a difference to care. She's over-invested.'

Karen looks over at the door and I push it open fully. The blood rushes up my neck.

'Chloe,' she says softly, 'I asked you to stay in our room,

didn't I? All okay?' She looks shocked, just for a second, but then her face returns to complete calm.

'The husband wants you back. Sorry. He wouldn't take no for an answer.'

'It's not safe for you to be out of that room,' she says. 'Another time, press the buzzer.' She holds my gaze and I know she really doesn't care if I've overheard. Her expression says that there's no doubt in her mind that she's right and she's doing me a favour by letting me know. I'm near tears. I excuse myself and tell her I'm going to the bathroom.

In the end cubicle, I sit on the lid, hands over my eyes.

'It's okay. It's not true. It's not true.' I whisper, over and over. I stop when I realise it's not helping.

I flush the loo, even though I haven't gone, and come out to find Dr Roshni is getting changed into scrubs and wellies. She must have heard me. She looks right through me and I think she's going to ignore me out of busy politeness, but before she turns to leave she gives me a brief, solid smile.

'Days like these you find out what you're made of,' she says.

'Yeah,' I say, but she's already swept off, an obstetric emergency far more important and also, probably, far easier to fix than a student midwife falling apart in the bathroom.

17

Examination

Friday, 27th July 2001

Today is the last of the first-year OSCEs exams. I drink my tea, unable to stomach coffee. Christopher points out this is a good sign, as having some nerves is important. He's hearty, telling me I'll do well. He thinks I'm just nervous and exhausted and soon I'll be back to normal, but I'm quiet and distracted over breakfast.

'And my parents are coming round for dinner. Something nice to look forward to,' he says.

Oh God. 'I almost forgot.'

'Don't worry. They'll love you. We're having lamb. Nothing for you to worry about. You just have to be here.'

I don't have the energy to be concerned right now, so I put it out of my mind.

I arrive at the skills lab early, with fifteen minutes to spend fretting. The corridor is golden, all lit up by the sun, and I wait in a plastic chair. I'm going to join Karen for one more day of placement, on Tuesday, after my written exam is done too. She'll decide whether I pass my placement then.

Two other students arrive. The older has wild eyes and tells me three times she got stuck in traffic and then couldn't find a parking space and thought she was going miss the exam. I smile weakly at her. I'm both agitated and weary as I look through my copy of *Skills for Midwifery Practice*.

An older male teacher in glasses, a shirt and a brown cardigan comes out of the office to tell us the rules. I don't know him, he's not from the midwifery department. *You must pass this exam to progress to the second year of your course. You must not ask the examiners for extra information.* We look at each other. *You must be in uniform with your name badge.* Well, you can see we all are and have.

I put my head in my hands, but neither of the other students pays attention. They're lost in their own individual bubbles of panic.

'Chloe Cawthorne?' It's Rosie who calls me in, and I have a wave of relief that it's her. She's in navy uniform, the first time I've ever seen her in one. She's very slender, a silver belt cutting her into an hourglass shape, her dreads twisted up in a butterfly clip. I'm glad it's Rosie, she'll be fair at the very least. At the sight of her, I want to blurt out everything.

I get up and all the blood rushes to my head and I feel nauseous and have that hot wave of saliva in my mouth that makes me think I'll have to run for it. But I clamp down on the feeling.

'Hey, Chloe. Don't you look nice in uniform?'

'Thanks. You too, actually.' I say and swallow.

Rosie waves me into the skills lab ahead of her. Two other lecturers are behind the desk. Adjoa is one of my favourites: she's a tiny Ghanaian woman with tight, fine cornrows, who researches diabetes in pregnancy and is always smiling. Sue, though, is a matron and a total hard ass.

'We record the exam so there's no query about your grade later,' Sue says, pointedly, without saying hello. 'Can you please look into the camera, and say your name, student number and date of birth?'

I do so, unable to relax my mouth, stuttering a bit. I hate this. I hate it.

The exam begins.

First I'm asked to do basic observations on a female dummy and it goes better than I thought possible. Sue keeps asking me why I'm doing things. I remember all the right words, diastolic, systolic, they trip off my tongue just like I know what I'm talking about.

Then I perform venipuncture on a fake arm, sterilising the area with a wipe, securing the tourniquet, the imitation blood a much lighter and redder colour than the real thing. After I've labelled the blood bottles clearly and handed them in for inspection, Sue says, 'The final question is a role play. Rosie will be the woman you're caring for...'

They get me to sit in a chair in front of the panel and though I manage to give them all eye contact, smiling, my heart starts trying to climb up my throat into my mouth.

'This client has arrived on labour ward at 4pm, five centimetres dilated, a primip. The pregnancy is unplanned and she is still unsure about becoming a mother. Discuss pain relief options with her.'

Sue is frowning. Panic hits the pit of my stomach and catches like a spark, spreading through my body. I look straight into the camera and then back at Rosie, who nods and smiles at me. I try and climb onto Rosie's calm and certainty like a raft.

'Um.'

'You have five minutes left, Chloe,' says Sue.

'Okay. Um. Hello.'

Sue writes something on her piece of paper and exhales loudly.

'Well, you could have a pool birth...'

Rosie leans towards me over the table, 'Sorry, what was your name?'

'That's prompting I'm afraid, Rosie,' Sue says loudly, staring at her.

'Sorry,' says Rosie, 'Carry on Chloe.'.

I close my eyes and will myself to imagine I'm in the birth centre. *You're pushing the door open. There she is, on the biggest day of her life. Your job is to help her find her feet. Whatever she needs is fine.*

'Hi,' I say, 'I'm Chloe. I'm a student midwife working here on labour ward. I'm sure my mentor will be coming along in just a moment, I've let her know you're here. What was your name?'

'Rosie. It's really hurting now, Chloe. I don't think I'm coping.'

I take a big breath, 'Okay. What about a bath? Have you tried water?'

'It's *really* hurting.'

'Okay, the pool might help.'

'Can't I have some drugs?'

'Yes. Gas and air?' I glance at Sue to try and see if I'm on the right track but she doesn't give me any eye contact. Then she says, 'Okay. Let's try something else. It's two hours later, and despite using gas and air, this client has been screaming through contractions for half an hour.'

Rosie raises her eyebrows and then settles her face again.

Don't panic. Don't panic, I think. I'm not listening to myself. I'm imagining Rosie finding out that the student in front of her is pregnant, is going to fail her placement, has screwed everything up.

'It's okay. It'll all be okay,' I say, 'You're doing really well. We can talk about an epidural if you like. The anaesthetist will need to come in.'

'I'm really scared of a big needle in my back.'

'Okay, well we can talk about the likelihood of anything going wrong, but it's a really small chance. An epidural would be totally your choice. The first thing we'd need to do is get you into a hospital gown and have a good listen to your baby to check they're coping well, because sometimes an epidural can worry them for just a little while. We tend to put a drip in your hand too, so we can give you fluids if you need them, is that okay? Do you have anyone with you to support you?'

'No! Whatever, just give it to me!'

'Okay. I'll call my mentor...'

'And that's time.' says Sue, looking at her watch.

'Thank you, Chloe.'

I'm shaking. Rosie looks at me with what I can only describe as pity.

I unlock the door, hoping for an empty flat, but Christopher's there in the living room marking essays, the flat filling with the smell of meat from the oven.

'Oh, hey. How did it go?'

'Awful,' I say, putting my keys on the hook. His eyes widen and I burst into tears.

'Oh – oh, no. Chloe.' he gets up and comes and hugs me into him, one cool hand on the back of my head. 'Hey, you poor thing. It'll be okay. I promise. Poor girl.'

'*I forgot fucking pethidine.*'

'What does that mean?'

'Pain relief options...'

'Oh. Well, you'll have learnt something. And you can do it again, right? It's only your first year, I bet it won't even count for your degree classification? My students can fail two whole modules.'

'Midwifery's different...'

He pulls me onto the sofa.

'Everything's going wrong,' I sob. 'I've fucked it all up. Sadie's birth... Dad... Karen hates me, she's probably going to fail me because she thinks I'm arrogant. Maybe I am. Maybe I'm a selfish, irresponsible, fucking arrogant person... and... I'm so screwed up...' I'm doubled over, crying, trying to get it out. He has no idea what I'm saying or why I'm so upset.

'Chloe. It'll be okay.'

He's trying to make light of it and distract me. My hair has fallen over my face and he parts it and kisses my neck.

'Try not to make one grade about your whole life. Everyone comes out of these things thinking they failed when they actually do alright. You're so bright. I look at these students I'm teaching and in comparison...'

I can't get any of it into words.

'You think you're responsible for all these women but you're just one person. And then your Dad and Ali... it's too much for anyone.'

I'm so tired of people telling me that I can't make a difference. He doesn't notice me stiffen.

He's trying to rock me, his forehead pressed into my shoulder, but I push him away.

'It's so hard. I think I can help, I really do. But I'm fighting all the time.'

He looks at me, head on one side. The sunlight is coming through the window, picking out every black speck and whirl in his grey eyes.

'I know your Mum was a midwife, but it's not the same as having experience, is it?' he says. 'Maybe she was a bit wild in what she believed, it sounds like that? Maybe that's why it's hard for you? Maybe just trust the qualified midwives for the moment, keep your head down more?'

I'm seething. 'But what about doing what the women want?' I say, through gritted teeth.

'Is this the epidural thing again? You like it when they have a normal birth, don't you? Was this what the question was on?'

'Kind of.'

'Aren't you forcing them *not* to have an epidural?'

'That's not what I said in the exam and that's never been what I've said to you!'

I get up and walk into the bedroom. I put my books, folders and one clean uniform into my bag. In the mirror, I look pale and terrified, though I feel furious. I wipe away the mascara which has trickled down under my eyes.

'Chloe?'

When I come back in Christopher is sat on the sofa looking tired and resigned.

'Are you going to the library? Are you revising? I don't think you're in any fit state to... Maybe just have a shower and get into something nice for when my parents come? These past few days I've noticed you've got lower and lower. You have to look after your mental health more. If you really want to look after women at work, you have to put yourself first...'

'*Fuck.*'

'Don't keep swearing.'

'I need to go and revise somewhere else.' I try to keep my voice level.

'Stay here. It'll be quieter. I can help if you like and then we'll have dinner.'

'No.'

'It would be much better to keep it calm, I can help by quizzing you –'

'Not this time,' I say. He gets up and leans on the breakfast bar.

'You know what Chloe, mostly, your life experience means you react with maturity and I'm so impressed with you. It's why I'm with you, right? But right now, this is teenage Chloe coming out.'

I want to kill him. I also want to tell him.

'Okay. Thanks.' I say flatly.

'Chloe –' he comes over and tries to put his arms around me. I push him away.

'Don't worry. It'll be alright. Go back to marking. It's good for me to know how you really feel.'

'Where are you going? Look, my parents won't mind if you're in a funny mood. They teach, they know what it's like, uni is a lot of pressure.'

'I'm going back to mine.'

'What?'

I turn back to him and though I know it's the most immature thing I could say it comes out anyway.

'I'll go where I want. I am so tired of people telling me what to do.'

I'm lying on my bed thinking.

When I was four or five, once Mum had finished the

midwifery work she set out to do in Alabama, we went travelling. I don't remember much. Wide-open meadows, being carried by Dad for some of the way when we went hiking. Craggy, snow-capped mountains in the distance and the smell of pine trees and cold water.

There's a photo in one of our family albums that I have a fuzzy memory of Mum taking. It's of a trail sign, clear green and white lettering telling us this is a high point, a separation of the major river systems. Raindrops falling to the left of the sign flow east towards the Atlantic Ocean. Raindrops falling to the right flow west, to the Pacific. A few centimetres landing difference means the drops will end up 2,000 miles apart.

Today, I feel like I'm standing on a continental divide.

I go downstairs, thinking about making a cup of tea. My boobs are swollen and my bladder is achy. There are a few dusty bottles of red wine that have been on top on the fridge for years and on an impulse, I open one. Dad's gone out, I'm not sure where. When he came in I told him I was back to revise and I nearly burst into tears. I told him I was begging him to keep his problems away from me until after my exams and his eyes widened, but he didn't say much. Later he disappeared with his backpack without explanation, whether to give me space or to keep out of trouble, I don't know.

I take the full glass back up to my room, the purple-black wine swishing around.

My midwifery posters that I put up during my A-levels look down at me. There's one of an eight-week fetus. They're ugly things, all limb buds and odd curves. They don't need to be pretty to be loved; they're safe and protected. I wonder if my baby looks specific to Christopher and me already, and then a cold feeling spreads from my stomach, up my back and into my chest. *This baby has a quarter of Mum's genes*, I realise.

I leave the wine where it is on my desk and instead pad back down to the kitchen to make camomile tea. I sit sipping it, flipping through my photocopied notes, nauseated and pretending to revise.

My finger is on an image of a cross-section of skin. *Epidermis. Stratum basale. Dermis.* I can't remember any of this. I'm going to fail this exam and I don't care. The lack of caring is bleak and awful, much worse than any pain or guilt or fear. I should be afraid to be in this house, given that the police could knock at any moment. But for some reason I'm not; it's like my room has gravitational pull. I need to be here.

I imagine coming home to Christopher's flat, pushing a buggy past the university as Noelia and everyone else qualifies.

I imagine being in this room with a baby, breastfeeding, bundling it up and leaving it in Dad's lap while I shower.

I put my head in my hands and cry and for a long time I can't stop. Eventually I get into bed again, wanting the soft pillow against my cheek, and I sleep and try not to dream but I do and there's Mum, alive in my bed, warm and I reach out to her and maybe there was a horrible mistake. I hug her hard enough for her to groan.

'Oof. That's a big cuddle, Chloe.'

I look again and she's cold as stone, her eyes staring. I was wrong, she's not alive after all.

My phone goes off and I'm glad of it, glad to be woken, and I think maybe I'm on call for Sadie and spring out of bed to get it from my bag in the corner of the room.

It's Christopher.

'Oh. Hey. What time is it?' I ask, confused.

'Five-ish. Where are you?' He sounds angry.

'I'm at Dad's.'

There's a silence.

'Can I come and pick you up? My parents are nearly here, dinner's at six.'

'Oh. Yeah. I don't think I can make it. Thank you, though.'

'Did you fall asleep?'

My voice is thick and confused.

'Just a power nap. I'm exhausted, it's all the revision.'

'Are you really going to miss tonight? Just because we had some stupid fight?'

'Christopher,' I interrupt him. 'I have reading week now and I need some time to think. Okay? Let me get through these few days. I promise we'll talk properly after that. But it's too much pressure otherwise.'

'Rubbish –'

'No, it's not. It's okay. I'm okay. Let me try and sort it all out. I'll do my best. It's all I can do.'

'You're being ridiculous.'

'I'm sorry.'

I hear the dial tone, he's put the phone down. I feel the weight and pressure of this responsibility and my love for Christopher, because I do love him and I love this baby and in another time and place this would have been my family. I close my eyes.

18

Leicester to London

Thursday, 2nd August 2001

I'm sitting in the delivery suite pool room, listening to Karen tell Rosie why she's not letting me pass this placement. This is my official end-of-year meeting with my personal tutor. Most of the other students have finished their placement already and just have the written exam to go before the three-week summer break.

'She's bright,' says Karen, 'But I can't in good conscience tick to say she takes safe direction at every turn at the moment. You know how big a responsibility this mentorship role is...'

Outside it's summer: ice-cream vans, people sipping from cans on the grass and kids with water pistols. In the birth room, it's cool with the windows and blinds closed, a small safe nest for a labouring woman. I'm sitting on a plastic stool, Rosie and Karen are up on chairs. I realise my shoulders are hunched so I pull myself together and sit up straight. The nausea is intense and there's pain that comes and goes. Part of me hopes this pain continues and part of me knows it won't.

I want to go home. Or I want to tell to Rosie to fight for me, to make this situation fair again. But I don't, I sit and listen.

'Chloe? Is there anything you want to ask?' says Rosie.

I don't think I've said a thing so far apart from 'Good morning'.

'No, I think I understand. I'll do a few more days with Karen, over at the birth centre in Melton Mowbray. And after that, we'll see.'

'Right. And you need to demonstrate to Karen that you're a perfectly safe student. I know you can do this.'

Rosie seems younger in a summer dress and boots today. Or maybe it's just because she's sat next to Karen. She looks at me with concern and I think back to asking for her permission to be Sadie's birth partner, seven months ago, in March, when I was so happy and confident, filled with joy at the prospect of being there for Sadie's birth.

'I'll do everything I can,' I say. 'I'll work the whole of August if I have to.'

'I don't think that's a good idea', says Karen, 'You're lucky I'm agreeing to getting these few days in, frankly. I've told Rosie I think you should just have the summer off and think about your choices. Repeating the year might be kinder for you, really, and you can work with me again. We'll really make sure you're safe. But we'll get these few shifts over with first if that's what we have to do,' says Karen briskly, 'Rosie, are we about finished? I need to go and put my lady on the monitor...'

'Yeah,' says Rosie, 'I'll just hang on to Chloe for a second if that's okay.'

Karen leaves without a backwards glance. I look at Rosie. Her dreads are flowing down her back and she looks like when I first saw her in the lecturers' office, tired but energetic, on my side, fierce about backing me up.

'Chloe. Why didn't you tell me about all this?'

I shrug.

'You're busy,' I say.

'It's what I'm here for. Is this why you looked so terrified in your OSCE?'

'I'm sorry.' I don't trust myself to talk too much.

'What are you sorry for?'

'Being a pain.'

'Chloe,' she says, leaning forward, 'You did come and tell me at the beginning of this placement that you had your concerns. That can be taken into account. I'd try and get you to work with another mentor, but legally, Karen's the one who has to sign you off right now, unless we make a formal complaint. That could take months, so it'd be almost certain you'd retake the year just for time reasons. I'm really sorry, I know it might not seem it, but this is the easiest path. I know you can do this.'

She looks worried though.

'I think I screwed my OSCE up too.'

She shakes her head.

'Rosie, it's okay. As hard as it is, if I have to drop down and do another year, I will. It's not a pride thing. If I'm off the course, so be it. I'm trying as hard as I can and I'll keep doing my best, trying to make the right choices. It's not like I ever had any guarantees, even with what I learnt from Mum, but… I'll make the most of it.'

I'm rambling now, unsure that this is the right thing to do but unable to stop. 'Because this is it, right? It's never straightforward. You just have to make the best decisions and then move on. And maybe that's what it's about, turning up every day and doing the best you can, making the most of the situation and getting it as right as possible for each woman, even when people tell you you're wrong.'

I'm nearly in tears. For a second I want to tell Rosie

everything and I think it's all going to come spilling out, but she puts one arm around me and hugs me, a brief, professional as possible squeeze. It stops me and I'm relieved, like I've been pushed out of the way of a speeding car. This is my problem alone and it's not fair to ask for help.

Friday, 3rd August 2001

As I join the crowd of students, I worry that I don't have any nerves about this exam. I am a fake, a fraud, floating above all this, it's all just sitting on the surface. I'm here staring at the vending machine chocolate, in the queue for the exam, knowing that after this is over I'm likely to care about the outcome, but today I can't seem to feel anything. I'm exhausted from thinking.

The Hawthorne Building entrance where we're queuing has a broad stone arch from the old city church in the entrance hall and they've encased it in a glass case like it's in a museum or something. We all line up next to it and I wonder how many women have stood next to these stones while praying for different circumstances.

Noelia finds me and says 'What's wrong with *you*?' by way of greeting.

'Morning,' I say to her.

'Darling, you look terrible. Did that boy keep you up all night?'

I smile, shrug and roll my eyes, thinking, *in a manner of speaking*.

'You're not nervous, are you?' she asks.

'Maybe a little bit. My OSCE was rubbish.'

She puts one hand on my shoulder. 'Me too. But exams

are so different from real life. Why haven't you been picking up your phone? We've all been revising together for reading week.' She means herself, Ada and Mehreen.

'Oh, you know. Working hard, keeping my head down.' I'm having a difficult time keeping the pain from my face.

'Shall we have coffee afterwards? You look like you need a chat.'

'Yeah,' I say. 'Let's get this over with, then.'

The line is moving into the exam hall. I don't like lying to Noelia, but I'll need to slip out early. There's no way I'm staying to talk to everyone in this cloud of detachment. And I'm not explaining now.

She's concerned, she scans me. 'Don't let it get under your skin, all this exam stuff. You're a good student, this is no problem for you... us oldies, on the other hand...'

I wish her luck and we take our seats and I stare out of the window into a deep blue sky. It's cloudless; it reminds me of the ocean and I want to lose myself in the colour.

The papers are handed out and I feel calmer than I've been in weeks. The concentration in the room is palpable and I fall into it like the flow of a river. I construct answers, check through and write in the details I've forgotten and here we go, of course, a question on pethidine, the opiate I forgot in the OSCE. I can do this, I can. I know the physiology, opioid receptors and the antidote, Narcan, in case it's needed, because pethidine can suppress breathing in babies who have received a dose through the placenta.

I run out of questions with 30 minutes left and stare out at the squirrels running across the grass and up into the trees. I think everyone else is still writing. I start to stress about having gone back to Christopher's to get some of my clothes and a few books. I'm not sure whether he will have noticed. I've done too much hurried packing this year.

The decision comes crashing back in, wave after wave, and it's making me sweat. I wipe my forehead with the sleeve of my jumper and hold my paper up in the air.

The examiner walks down between the tables and takes it from me and I feel eyes on me as I leave. In the entrance I gently pat the glass case of the polished stones and wonder if Mum ever did the same when she was at uni and what mindset she was in, and I'm desperate to slip through a hole in time and ask her, but this is real life and I just walk home in the sun to wait for tomorrow.

Saturday, 4th August 2001

I've packed my portable CD player, with Massive Attack and the Red Hot Chili Peppers and also the Hugh Masekela album from Mum's collection, for something lighter. I have my placement notes and a few of Ali's stupid fashion magazines in case I can't concentrate, some pads, paracetamol and my wash stuff. I'll be gone for 48 hours or so.

I've found somewhere to stay with one of Ali's friends who lives in Brixton. Christopher keeps texting and I reply to maybe one out of five, but I'm running out of credit. I don't want to call him.

My phone beeps while I'm walking. It's a message from him.

Sweetheart, when are you coming home? Having dinner with supervisor and others from uni – wondered if you wanted to come?

I text back: *Conference, out of town. Tlk soon.*

At the train station, the woman behind the counter is squat and cheerful. She says, 'Alright m'duck? Cheer up, might never happen,' and I force myself to smile. I wonder if she's ever been through anything similar.

On the train I sit and stare, thick gold wheat filling the view through the windows. It's warm even at just past seven in the morning and I have the same horrible, tortuous nausea I've had for days.

I couldn't face eating anything so early and I can smell urine from the toilets really badly. I get my mirror out and check my makeup and reapply a bit of foundation and eyeliner. The train is full and a blond guy in black jeans smiles at me and I think *you don't know what you'd be getting yourself into* and turn away.

I listen to Massive Attack for a few tracks but it's totally the wrong choice. I put on Hugh Masekela and close my eyes. I feel like Mum is sitting across from me listening to the African music. She always wanted to work in Africa. I think the last time I heard this album Mum didn't even have a diagnosis of high blood pressure and she was spring cleaning. I can nearly hear her singing, waving her bum in the air as she cleaned the fridge on her hands and knees.

The album finishes and the white noise of the train is comforting and I lose myself in the woodland and towns out of the window.

The GP gave me a leaflet with a map. The decision to come to here was because they offer weekend appointments, but, more importantly, here I'm anonymous. I can't risk seeing anyone at the Royal. At King's Cross I join the Underground, then I get off at Warren Street and walk until I find the road and the Marie Stopes sign.

The inside of the clinic isn't that nice; it has plastic chairs and scuffed white walls. The receptionist is young and in a flowery top, filing beige folders. I give her my details and take a seat, wrapping my arms around myself.

I look more carefully. Despite it being run down, someone has tried to make the waiting room welcoming. A tank has a few ugly goldfish swimming in it, there are a few plants and the radio is quietly playing Shania Twain.

The waiting room is full even though it's early. There's a black girl with golden highlights, her boyfriend with his cap on backwards, both glaring, a Middle Eastern-looking guy with acne who can't be more than 14, insecure and wiry. A young Chinese girl with straight hair and glasses looks exhausted. I try to think about how lucky we all are to be here.

This isn't so bad. There's nothing to worry about. I'll be back home in no time.

'Would you like a chaperone while I do this scan? Someone else in with us?'

'Oh...no, I'm sure it'll be fine.'

'And it says here you were taking the pill?'

'Yes.'

'Any missed pills?'

'I... I don't know. Maybe once. I've been... busy.'

'Okay. Can you lie on the couch please?'

I look up at the ceiling as I unbutton my jeans and cover the top of them with folded blue tissue to protect them from the ultrasound jelly, which is cold enough to make me jump. The foam ceiling tiles are in poor condition, white and cracked, with some missing.

'Would you prefer me to keep this screen turned away?'

'Yeah.'

He's silent for a few minutes, moving the probe this way and that.

'Would you like to know whether it's twins or not? And the gestation?'

'Um. Yes please.'

'Ok. I can see it's a singleton pregnancy. And I believe' he clicks something on the probe, 'you're about ten weeks.'

It's older than I was hoping for and I am glad that these days I am sure there is no God. We have to do the best we can with the cards we have been dealt, that's what Mum would have said. She was an atheist really, with hippy stuff here and there. She believed the right choice was whatever was right for the woman.

'Can I get you a tissue?' I blink and I realise my face is wet with tears. I nod and the sonographer hands me some hand towels, which are scratchy under my eyes.

'Are you seeing the counsellor today?'

'I don't know. Sorry. It doesn't matter. I've made my decision.' He's finished and I wipe myself clean, pull my jeans up and button them again.

'Okay, well we can start that process for you today with one set of tablets you'll swallow. Then you'll come back tomorrow for the next set,' he says. He's a huge black guy with cornrows who's looking at me with such unguarded compassion that it makes me cry even harder. The tears are streaming down my face and my shoulders are shaking, 'But see the counsellor anyway. Talk it through, yeah?' He has a low voice like gravel and a South London accent.

I'm so all over the place and he's calmly wiping gel off the probe and filling in notes, some technical middle-aged man who must see silly little girls like me all the time.

'I just don't want to hurt anyone.' I hear myself say. He keeps writing, but his response is so empathetic that in years to come I'll look back on this moment and wonder whether I

240 • NEW WALK

made it up or embellished it.

'Far more important that you don't hurt yourself. Look, this is why it's so hard,' he says, 'Your job is to choose as best you can and then respect yourself for that decision.'

He puts the pen down and takes me through to see the counsellor. She's brilliant, but really I don't need anything more than that.

Sunday, 5th August 2001

I'm given a small plastic medicine cup containing the second lot of tablets that will start the cramps.

The nurse says, 'You'll need to put these as high up into your vagina as possible. Legally you need to do this here, as you can't take them off site. And Chloe, you're on your own in the bathroom when you give them to yourself. Are you heading back to Leicester on the train today? The tube and the train back home?'

'Yes.'

'Let me show you where the bathroom is. There are some sample bags in there. If someone happened to be taking something out of the clinic, I'd suggest using one of those.'

She looks at me with a bright expression.

'All right?'

We are two women breaking rules together and I'm very grateful to her. But more than that there's something about the suggestion that makes me realise she respects me, and this makes all the difference in the world.

19

Still Life

When I get off the train in Leicester, it's about 2pm, a Sunday afternoon with a white sky and muggy air. I walk home and when I open the front door and call 'Dad?' there's no response.

I go upstairs and check his room, which is littered with plates and tobacco. He's out. I offer up a silent prayer of thanks for this, to anyone listening.

I glance at the ceiling in his room. I've crammed any thoughts about this away. I'm tired, not thinking straight, but I don't have any other options.

Once I've unpacked, I go straight to the bathroom and shake the tablets out of the bag and onto my hand. There are four of them. They are hexagonal, white and each slightly smaller than a five-pence piece.

I push the tablets high into my vagina and put a pad on. I am still calm and decided. I hope it lasts. There are other things I need to get done in this calm way. I unpack my bag and drink down a glass of wine. Alcohol would have been the drug of choice for most women, historically. I don't want to take paracetamol, I want to experience this as it should be. That might be a little strange, but I'm okay with that.

Then I sit on my bed and call Christopher. He answers after two rings.

'Hey. It's me.'

'Hello.' He sounds offbeat and unlike himself. 'How was the exam? And the conference?'

'Uh... the exam was okay, I think. It's done, anyway. The rest of the weekend has been... alright.'

'Yeah?'

I ask him about his weekend and he answers vaguely. The wine is helping. I'm not lying, not really, I'm just leaving things out for now. It's all for the best.

'Can I pick you up in the car in a bit? We could go and see a film.'

'I just need to sort something.'

'Not a horror flick. Something else. Or there's a party tonight if you fancy it.'

'As I said, I need to get some stuff sorted first.'

'Can I help?'

'Oh, no. Don't worry. Go to the party, really, I don't mind.' There's a silence.

'Right. I guess I'll get on then,' I say. I'm not sure whether or not I feel the first stretch and pressure of a cramp already. I could be imagining it.

'Go and make the most of your Sunday night,' I tell him. There's a long silence.

'It won't be much fun without you,' he replies.

'That's sweet. Right, I should get on.'

After we hang up I exhale and sit for a long moment.

Then I put the TV on in my room and it's *Dad's Army*, which I'm happy about, I often watch it with Nanna. *Don't panic, Captain Mainwaring.* The feelings are building, tugging at me now, relentless and impossible to ignore. But I do try and ignore it. It's what I'd tell a woman I was caring for to try and do.

I take down a box that I've kept that's full of Mum's stuff, old perfume bottles, one purple crystal earring (the other long lost), cinema tickets from when we went to see *Titanic*. There's a cashmere scarf with purple flowers and an old Gold Coco Chanel box in there and I leave them out on my desk.

The cramps begin to come and go like the tide and I plug in my electric blanket and put it on my back and watch Pike singing at the German soldiers about Hitler being a berk.

The episode ends and when I get up to turn the channel over, there's a gush and I go to the bathroom. When I pull my underwear down it's not blood like I expected, but a small amount of clear fluid. I know it, it's bleachy and bodily and it's weird, but it smells a lot like semen, from the hormones. It's the waters around the baby that have gone and this is a shock. I wonder if I was further along than they thought. I put my head in my hands and stay put on the loo. The cramps are unbelievable, much more painful than I was expecting, and I'm hot and clammy.

After fifteen minutes of this, the toilet seat starts to dig in and I put a fresh pad on and go back to my room just in my knickers and top. This is pretty awful. I lie on my side on the bed and I'm glad for all the tiny acts of patience I've given women, because I'd be feeling like this was punishment for my lack of empathy otherwise.

There's another gush and this time I can tell it's blood from the sticky feeling. Actually, *shit* it's gone through my pad and underwear onto the duvet. In between cramps I manage to strip the bed and put the sheets into the bath to soak and I run the cold tap. The sheets billow and roll like sails and the seconds when I'm not cramping are a wonderful relief.

I go back to my room and put on some fresh underwear, black this time, and a pad and a black pair of shorts in case I bleed through again. I lie on my side on a dark blue bathroom towel.

The pain is deep inside my pelvis, radiating out through my back and I press my hand into it. I am so glad this isn't happening on the train, and I'm amazed that being in public while this is going on must be a possibility for some women, whether they're having a miscarriage or a termination. I don't know how I'd cope. The TV is still on: it rattles through *The Simpsons* and on to the news.

Then the wine has worn off, it's evening and everything is intense. There's been a train crash in France and I'm sad about this and the pain combines with this feeling.

The pain encircles me and I start to shake. The feeling is moving downwards and pressure is building and building and I know this is it. I feel something in my vagina and pull my underwear down and there's a tennis ball-sized clot of tissue that I pull away and I know at once that this is the baby. I leave it on the towel.

I feel better immediately, the relief is thick as oxygen. I pull my underwear back up and sit and cry and shudder, but it's okay. I wrap my arms around myself. I'm proud. I've done it.

In the bathroom I squeeze the water out of the sheets and put them in the washing basket and put my stained underwear in the bin. They're too far gone.

Then I shower and get changed into my cords and a clean top. I'm okay. Thank God I live in a country where I can be okay.

I look at the lump of tissue. The thought of flushing it

away is horrific.

I wrap it gently in the cashmere scarf and put it inside the gold perfume box.

I make a cup of tea and sit at the kitchen table and I'm hit by the speed of everything that's happened. Not just with this situation, but from the moment Mum died. It feels like everything since then has happened on fast-forward. It's surreal.

Mum wasn't religious, but she did like rituals. Lighting candles for making wishes, magical Christmas gingerbread, everyone had to come to the seaside and paddle and wash their face in the salt water at least once a year, even if it was cold enough to turn your lips blue.

I put my boots on and go into the shed to find the spade. It's chaos in there, rolling papers among the wood chips and old cups of tea with rotting mould around the edges. Dad used to keep all his tools on a board with their outlines showing where they hung, but now they're slung anywhere.

I dig right at the edge of the garden, under the sloping grey tree with the thick bark. The earth is hard: the sun has dried it out and there are lots of stones, so it takes a while to make it a deep hole, half a metre or so to stop animals. I try to be fast. I'm worried about Dad coming home and having to explain myself.

The sun is shining through the old raspberry canes and the flowers that Mum planted and I can see the sunflowers in pots next door through the fence. The sky has changed to being a light blue; it looks more like a dawn sky than an evening one. I think about Nanna. She'd spend time enriching this soil. She's always telling me that the earth in her garden is fine and easy to dig because it's been looked after with years of compost and growing beans and peas. What would she say if she knew a potential great-grandchild was under the earth in her daughter's garden?

When the hole is dug I stand for a minute. I can hear pigeons cooing in the tree and kids playing in the road outside.

I say, 'I'm sorry. You would have been wonderful. I hope you understand.'

I put the box in the hole and cover it with earth, ten, eleven, twelve shovelfuls, and pat it down.

I close my eyes and I can see the yellow and green light of the garden shining through my eyelids. This is my own ritual.

20

Enid's Care

Thursday, 9th August 2001

It's 6.45 in the morning when I arrive for my first shift with Karen at St Mary's birth centre. I'm feeling determined, but a bit cut off from everything. I'm still bleeding, more than I thought, heavier than a normal period. And the cramps are pretty bad.

This is a beautiful old stone hospital building, with just two labour rooms and eight postnatal beds. It's in the tiny town of Melton Mowbray, which is a bit rough in places but basically quite nice, and has a whole economy based around making pork pies. In other circumstances I'd be excited about working at St Mary's. It has a fantastic reputation. Lots of women have their babies at the bigger hospitals and then transfer back just to stay in the postnatal ward because the care is that good.

I'm early and there's no one around, but I answer a buzzer anyway, following the signs to the postnatal bay and washing my hands. I help a mum with a pink nightie who looks at the end of her tether to latch on her daughter, who is screaming loudly enough to wake all the other mothers in the bays. She just needed to be a bit quicker when the baby opened her mouth, but she's clearly tried this process about fifty times already so I tell her she's doing amazingly and to press the buzzer again if there's a problem. The baby is now sucking with full cheeks.

Then I make a coffee in the hospital kitchen. I'm not sleepy, but I'm also not taking any chances – I need to be sharp. The Melton Mowbray midwives who have been on the night shift are in with a lady who's labouring in the pool, so I sit on my own in the office for a bit, sipping my drink and thinking about how today might go.

At five to seven, I'm surprised by Enid walking in, in her usual black skirt and cardigan, crucifix and lanyard. I assume she's just here for a meeting or something, but when I say good morning and ask her what she's up to she says 'I do work on the shop floor from time to time, you know, young Chloe, to keep my eye in. Maybe we'll work together for a bit, if your mother is happy,' and I rush to say that would be wonderful, though I doubt Karen will agree.

Even through my haze of anxiety about today and my awkwardness in talking to her, I do love her Irish accent. It's so comforting, soft as down. She sits down heavily and doesn't say anything more.

Being here at this time of year can't be covered up. Only students who have lost time through sickness or who need remedial hours will be around. I wonder if Enid knew about me being given extra time for this placement already.

To break the silence I ask her if she wants a cup of tea. She agrees and I go and make it. As it brews, I stare out of the window into the tiny hospital garden with an apple tree in the centre, daisies and dandelions thick in the grass.

It's at this moment that my mind chooses to take inventory. I still haven't looked in the attic, I can't bring myself to. It's a massive risk, on top of everything else, but I think Dad's trying to be respectful. At least none of his stoner mates have been around since I arrived again. I'm putting all my effort into ignoring the situation until after... after I know what will happen, with everything. I wonder what on earth Enid would think of my messy home life this year.

But Dad looks better; he's paying more attention to how he's dressing and he's shaving again and he's even had a haircut. And I think he's clearing some of the stuff in the garden away. I saw him put a few bin bags in the car to take to the tip.

I think about Christopher. Christopher sends me one text every night, always the same thing.

Let me know when you're coming back.

And there've been some texts from Ali.

Chlo, bmpd in2 Chris. Hes weird. Whts gng on? Xx

I texted back: *Nothing, just at Dad's to revise better. Talk soon xx*

A few hours later she replied:

B careful. Ask hm wht up with hm xx

What do you mean? xx

Jst ask xx

I bring the tea back to the office, where one other younger midwife is now seated at the table and Enid is answering the phone.

'Good morning, midwife speaking. Oh yes. No, I'm sure we'll be alright. Not a heavy workload today. I'll take your student out on community with me. You feel better now. Thanks for letting us know.'

She looks at me.

'Your mentor's Karen Hodgson, yes? She's off sick today. Are you supposed to be working 12 hours? We'll work together all day then.'

I thank her and make sure I come across as happy, which under any other circumstances I would be. I think Enid's an amazing midwife.

I'm in charge of the A-Z map as Enid drives and I'm flicking through, but Enid seems to know the whole of Rutland by heart anyway. I wonder how many hours she's spent on these roads. I know she was a community midwife for more than a decade.

'You're coming up to the end of your first year,' says Enid, 'How have you been finding it?'

I have no idea how much she knows. I decide to skirt around the issue.

'Oh, you know. Wonderful. Challenging.'

'Mm hm, sounds about right.'

Just like when I was on the train to London, wheat fields line the windows. It's a perfectly still and sunny morning.

'Anything about the challenges you'd like to share with me?'

'Um...'

I consider for a second, unable to put it into words. Part of me wants to ask for advice. I'd especially like to know what Enid thinks Mum would have done in this situation, if she has any insight there. But my confidence is paper thin and I don't want to come across as critical of Karen.

'Ask Karen Hodgson for *actionable* feedback then,' she says. 'She's a very experienced mentor.'

'Yes – I know,' I say miserably. 'Thank you.'

Then she surprises me by saying, 'You're notorious for that pinard, you know. Not many students bother. Keep on using it.'

Her phone goes off. It's a high-pitched, horrible tune; I've noticed a rule with phones, the more important the professional, the sillier their ring tone is. Dr Roshni's is always going off with a sort of 'huluhoo huhoo' noise.

'Can you answer that for me?'

Enid's bag is next to my feet and I scrabble for it.

It's the community office: one of the ladies booked for a home birth is in labour. The midwife asks if we'd like to take her, as we're close by and the couple don't mind having a student. The on-call midwife can come in to take over the community visits.

'What fun! And how considerate, starting to labour at the beginning of the day, not the end.' Enid has lit up, smiling.

For a second, she reminds me of my Mum, the excitement on her face when she was on her way to a birth. Enid cuts into my thoughts.

'Have you ever done a home birth before?'

'Just one,' I say and then realise that's sort of a lie. The home birth I saw was in America, and it's not like I was giving any care aged four.

'And did you get this couple's names?'

'Oh, just mum's name, Dawn Howell! And the address and phone number. Sorry, I didn't get the dad's name.'

Enid shakes her head and flicks the indicator on to turn off the field road; she must know a back route.

'It's always a good idea to get a proper handover on the phone. The midwife should have known really. You got her parity, but a quick rundown of what happened last birth wouldn't have gone amiss... anyway, not to worry. There'll be names on the home birth list in my diary, the folded yellow piece of paper...'

My heart sinks. I have the overwhelming feeling of not being able to do anything right.

'Okay,' I say, 'Thank you.'

We're silent again until Enid asks me to direct her and we find our way through a maze of back streets to Dalby Road. The houses are big with bay windows and thick sash curtains.

As we're getting all the stuff out of the back of the Beetle, a tiny, wiry, springy guy with short-cropped brown hair opens the door and waves. He's smiling, tense and electric, rocking on his feet, while we take the resus equipment and labour kit out of the car. He's wearing blue jeans and a navy top and he stands to one side to let us in.

'Hi! Hullo. Come on in. She's in the bedroom. I kept asking if we should go downstairs, the room's all set up for her, but she won't say much.'

Enid shoots me a significant look. The guy is already disappearing up the stairs, which twist around the corner after a few steps. Still in our jackets and me with my placement backpack and Enid with the home birth kit in an old fashioned doctor's bag, we follow him up two flights.

In the bedroom, Dawn is in the corner of a huge bed with a cream, flowered throw, in a room with strange, slanting angles in the ceiling, right at the top of the house. The room is spotless with cream carpets and there's a wooden chest at the base of the bed and a small red sofa with cushions that look like they may have been homemade, by someone very good at that kind of thing.

Dawn, like her husband, is petite. She has a huge bump and in her position on her hands and knees I can see the muscles in her arms and shoulders. She's wearing a black crop top and billowing cloth trousers and she has her forehead on the pillow, chanting, 'C'mon baby, c'mon baby, c'mon baby...'

When she finishes her contraction she looks around at us.

'Sorry. I'm waving my behind at you,' she murmurs and we all laugh. Her husband keeps laughing for longer than us and then goes and crouches next to her.

'You alright?'

'Yes, Simon,' she says, 'I've done it before, remember. Have you offered these two a drink?'

'Oh, you don't need to worry about us.' Enid is looking through her diary, She introduces both of us and then says, 'Dawn, this might not be the best place to have a baby. Too many soft furnishings. We can do things anywhere you like, but also, if we needed to get down the stairs in a hurry, you see where I'm going with this...'

'Yes... I know... came up for a nap and I got stuck on the bed,' she replies. 'We need to go down...'

'Downstairs is all set up with the shower curtain,' Simon says, proudly, 'And all her other stuff. Shall we?'

Dawn smiles, closes her eyes and starts to contract again. I'm in the corner of the room, trying not to draw attention to myself or disturb Dawn, but Enid beckons me over. Enid has found Dawn's hand-held pregnancy notes on the dresser and is flicking through.

Enid looks huge in this room, but she also sort of fits. She looks capable. I look at her and know her calm and solid confidence is something I want to have one day. If I ever get through this.

'So tell me what you'd do now, Chloe. While we're waiting for Dawn...'

Simon has one hand on Dawn's back and I can tell he's listening to me too. *Like a lamb to the slaughter*, I think.

I whisper, 'I'd do obs. Blood pressure, pulse, temp. I'd do a palpation. I'd ask about baby's movements and the colour of the liquid if Dawn's waters have gone. I'd listen in and offer a vaginal examination.'

Enid opens her eyes wide and nods.

'Hmm. Carry on then. You're in charge,' she says.

'You waters haven't gone, have they love?' says Simon, prompting, 'And this baby's been kicking all night, hasn't it?'

Dawn stops contracting and I go and crouch next to the bed. She looks over at me, as does Simon. With his spiky hair, brown eyes and wary expression he makes me think of a fox.

'Hey Dawn,' I say. She smiles and I keep my voice gentle and quiet, remembering what Mum once referred to as 'vocal anaesthesia'.

'We usually ask to do some checks to see if you and baby are okay. And at some point Enid,' I nod towards her, 'will call a second midwife so she has another pair of hands at the birth. It's sort of difficult to know when that might be without doing an examination, a vaginal examination, but it's totally your choice if you want one or not.'

Dawn nods, her expression cloudy. I don't think she's really heard me until she says,

'Let's get downstairs now. I don't think it's going to be too long.'

Simon runs his hand through his hair, 'Darling, you said that last time, for hours.'

'Yes... that's true... but...'

She dips her head again and starts contracting. She makes a huge noise, a mouth-open, working noise. I can hear her pain, but there's also an undercurrent of comfort there. There's an element of sex to it and I remember it's all the same hormones working on her body. Oxytocin is the hormone of love, endorphins are for pleasure, noradrenaline provides energy, and these are all part of labour.

I look at Enid and smile with urgency, knowing we need to get Dawn downstairs sharpish. When Dawn's contraction has finished, Enid and I help her move in a three-person dance, stopping when she stops, Simon having run down ahead.

Down in the lounge, Simon has set up flickering candles on the marble mantelpiece, the curtains are drawn and the blue carpet is covered in thick opaque plastic. The sofa is covered with a thinner plastic sheet and a towel and I also put a blue absorbent pad under Dawn's bum as she lies down, just in case her waters go.

First, I try to do a palpation, though I know I only have the beginning of this skill and Dawn's skin, tiger-striped with stretch marks and divided by a brown linea nigra from the top of her bump to just above her pelvis, yields lumps and bumps that I can't map. Then I think I find it, a continuous curve, the baby's back and the soft roundness at the top of her belly that must be the bum.

Simon's hovering by me, 'Chloe, what causes that? The brown line? We were talking about it, weren't we love?' Dawn doesn't answer, her eyes are half closed.

'Oh, it's hormonal,' I say, absently. 'You get a big flood of hormones to do with melatonin production in baby, I think, Enid, is that right? It might be ROA, by the way, can you check?' I look at Simon, 'That means Right Occipito Anterior. I think baby's back's on this side,' I gesture to my left, Dawn's right.

Enid puts down the notes she was reading and comes to repeat what I just did and nods briskly after a few seconds,

'Yes. ROA. And the head is really down, I can barely feel it. It's all normal. And yes, she's right about melatonin.'

'Good! Great!' says Simon and I have to smile at his enthusiasm. I have to stop myself from catching his jumpiness though. Slow and steady is right for labour, but I'm second-guessing everything because I have a horrible fear that Enid's going to turn to me in the car and say *I was wrong. I shouldn't have invited you to the interview last year. This is not the career for you.*

I tell myself to not fall prey to those kind of thoughts and bring myself back to the moment. I have a listen in with the sonicaid and the heart rate sounds beautiful, 135 beats per minute, relaxed and happy.

'So were you wanting an examination, Dawn?' I say, glancing at Enid to see her reaction, but she's shaking her head.

'I'm not sure I'd do one, Chloe. I think I'll call our backup. This is a normal mum, normal birth last time and she's starting to bear down.'

I turn back to Dawn.

'What would you like to do?' I ask.

'No examination... stay here for a moment. Rest,' she says.

'Okay,' I say, smiling and sitting back on my heels. Enid is on the phone ringing the community office to call the second midwife.

I realise my pinard is in my bag by my feet.

'Dawn, I've got my Mum's pinard with me. Would you mind me having a quick listen in with it?' *Damn*. I didn't mean to say it was Mum's, it's not a conversation that needs to be had right now. Enid's eyes flicker towards me. I see Simon turn his head in interest too.

'Oh, yeah, sure, I've heard of them,' says Dawn, 'Okay,

while there's not a contraction coming...'

I get it, taking it out of the cloth bag. I position it over where I found the baby's heartbeat with the sonicaid. I put my ear over it and take my hands away so I'm keeping it in place just from the weight of my head. For a second I can't hear anything but the movement of my hair against my ear. Then I tune in and there it is, the vibration of the heartbeat in the distance, a tiny flutter.

I listen for about fifteen seconds and count 38 beats, but I can feel Dawn wanting to move and so I let her go. I can see Enid out of the corner of my eye setting up the resus equipment.

Dawn wants to get up and hold onto the back of the sofa, so I help her into that position. Simon has turned on some music on the CD player, some violins and piano. It's lovely and I think about how this scene could not be any more different than waiting for the sound of the ambulance siren at Sam's.

Then Dawn moves over to the doorway, bracing her hands on either side of the frame. She gives a huge guttural grunt and starts to cry out, her legs apart. I look at Enid, unsure what to do, thinking we should probably help Dawn take off her trousers because I'm not sure how fast this will go, but Enid keeps working, testing the bag and mask.

'Dawn, is this baby coming now?'

'Maybe!' she says, in a long, thin grinding voice and then 'OH!' and she then screams, long and hard and Simon freezes. The noise is of an ungodly volume, she's howling and then she stops, panting.

'Is this okay?' she asks, and Enid says, in a voice of total calm, 'If you want to have a baby, it's just fine. Simon, could you help Dawn with her trousers. And Chloe, I think you should put some gloves on.'

I nod and grab some from the pile of equipment Enid's left out. Dawn is now totally naked. She seems to want to stay standing in the doorway, so I leave her where she is, covering the floor with inco pads under her, thinking Enid will tell me if I'm doing anything wrong. My heart is still in my mouth.

'Can I listen in, Dawn? Just a quick one?' I ask, wanting to know what the baby's heart rate is.

'Yeah,' she gasps, but then she starts to scream again and waters burst over her legs. It's a clear, pink-tinged colour and I scrabble to try and listen in, but Dawn bats my hands away.

Enid is there next to me, with a towel, and Simon is there too and I'm not sure what to do. I need to listen to the baby's heart rate, otherwise it's unsafe care. I look at Enid but she's giving nothing away. And then I realise that her backup is not going to make it on time, it's just us two.

Dawn dips her knees and says, *'Oh God, oh God...'* and because there's no contraction, I try and listen again with the wand of the sonicaid. I can't hear anything, it's all just crackling and I look at Enid and she says, 'It's probably too low,' and then I almost see all of Dawn's energy going downwards and I can glimpse the baby's head, under pressure with wrinkles and dark hair, balled up against Dawn's perineum.

'Okay, vertex visible at 11.44...' says Enid, still in a voice of total calm, and then with another tremendous scream the baby's head is born and Dawn reaches backwards to cup it. I move forward and hover but she's got it, the baby is born and she moves one hand forward to catch then goes down on her knees, the baby pink, cross and bawling in her arms.

Dawn brings the baby to her chest and Enid covers it with a towel. I haven't had to do anything and I look at Enid, concerned I missed something, but she just smiles at Dawn and says, 'What did you get?'

Dawn takes a big shuddering breath. 'Oh sweetheart... Hello baby. Si, we got a girl!'

Simon has wet cheeks and is crying openly. He puts his face up to Dawn's. At some point, he's put glasses on and he looks much younger and far more vulnerable. Even through my relief and delight, the noise shocks me, because I don't think I've ever seen a guy cry like that, not even Dad.

And then I take a few breaths to compose myself and I have the realisation that this is the most privileged place I could be in. Not just for this couple, but for Sadie and Sam and all the others. Perhaps Sam most of all, in many ways.

Enid says, 'Congratulations, you two. Let's put a clean, dry towel over baby. C'mon Chloe...'

I help Dawn onto the sofa and get Simon a cushion so he can kneel beside his daughter and his wife, and sit in the background, watching them together.

21

Results

Tuesday, 21st August 2001

I'm in the queue at student services. I'm surprised that it's open after the end of term, but the summer school is running and by the sound of things the others who are picking up their grades are language students over from France. The line is moving slowly and I'm impatient.

In the end, in the stuffy little community office where my final assessment took place, Karen signed me off with no debate. She moved quickly, seamlessly ticking the boxes and signing in a rush, like it was all inconsequential.

Then she left the room without looking at either me or Rosie, muttering something about *friends in high places,* which I couldn't work out.

Rosie leant forward and said, 'That home birth with Enid? She was very impressed with you, Chloe. She said it was more like working with a second or third-year. She's made a point of telling Karen and me that.'

It took a moment to sink in.

'But she never said anything to me! I had no idea she thought that!'

'Yeah, well, Enid's a bit like that, isn't she? I don't think I've ever heard her compliment anyone face to face. But I don't think Karen would have failed you, anyway. You know what you're doing.'

'Then what was Karen trying to do?'

Rosie starts talking before I've finished the question.

'Chloe, you have to realise where Karen's coming from and how's she's been trained. How hard we all have to work to get these women through safely. She's looked after a heck of a lot of clients and now care's changing. That must be very difficult for her. We'll be speaking to her about her... um, mentoring style, but she definitely wouldn't have signed you off unless she was happy you were safe. And you'll have done her some good too.' Then she adds, 'Probably best not to mention that to her in so many words...'

I'd still be walking on air now except for the little matter of my OSCE result. Right now I'm getting stared at by the glacial and beautiful French girls with their satchels and long eyelashes, who might think I'm a bit weird. I probably do look like I've just stepped out of a wind tunnel given the few weeks I've just had, though they could be blinking a bit at the De Montford University gospel choir, which you can hear loud and clear across the road from the Portland Building because every window is open. I don't know what they're singing but it's gorgeous, lots of enthusiastic part harmonies and sweeping high solos.

Eventually the students clear and the woman behind the counter smiles at me, 'Is this it m'duck?' she asks, 'Your final grade for the year? There's only a few of you left from your cohort to come and get them, yes, let me see, here we are...'

I'm handed an A5 brown envelope labelled with my name and student number. I thank her and stand in the corridor to open it. Then I put it into my backpack and walk home.

I put my keys in the bowl and then sink into a kitchen chair. The house is quiet and I consider getting up and making some coffee and finding the biscuits, but I can't be bothered. I can do everything at my own pace now, no pressure. I can hear the hum of the fridge and music coming from the garden and some banging and sawing coming from the shed.

I go outside. Helga is in the grass at the bottom of the garden. I watch her wiggling her bum before she pounces on something, but she misses and stalks off, annoyed. I can see Dad through the spiderwebbed window of the shed, his pale face staring down at whatever he's working on. I watch him for a few seconds. He's focused and hasn't seen me.

'Dad?'

His expression changes as he hears me and looks up and opens the door. He's dazed, his mind still in work mode, wiping his sawdusty hands on his black jeans.

'I've done it!' I wave my grade slip at him.

'Great,' he says, elated, 'Well done! Amazing! Fucking well done, knew you'd do it!' Then he pulls back and looks confused, 'No – hang on, you've done what?'

I laugh and hand him the piece of paper.

'I got through my first year of uni. In fact, it's better than that. I got 71 per cent across the board, that's a first.' I look over his shoulder at the list of grades, 'I thought that couldn't possibly be right with the extra time I needed for this placement, but look, it's there in black and white. I can even see where they've put in the extra days I had to do... and my OSCE, that's the practical exam, I got 60 per cent in that, so not brilliant, but all my essay grades pull it up...'

'Amazing!' he says again.

He studies the paper. The music is playing on his shed sound system, it's Led Zepplin. I know the song, it's *The Rain*.

'I'm going to make us dinner tonight... I'll make a ruby... and I'll call Ali...!' He rushes into the house, sawdust falling off him, still holding onto my grade slip. I go into the shed, turn the music off, shut the door and then follow him, grinning.

In the kitchen, he's got his apron on and he's getting out the saucepans. I've no idea what he's going to cook, I don't think we've got that much in. For a horrible second I think we've got mice again, but then I realise he's just spilt black rice all over the kitchen side. When he sees I'm in the kitchen too he points at me with both forefingers, like he's just remembered something.

'Chloe, I need to show you this.'

I don't reply.

'I didn't want to bother you, you've been working so hard. But it's getting silly.'

Still in his apron, he goes up the stairs. I stand uncomfortably, not wanting to follow. The happiness of this day could be ruined by having to acknowledge that we still have this huge problem. But maybe addressing it now is the responsible thing to do. I can't pretend I'm not living with a drug dealer anymore.

Going back to Christopher's, if I decide to do that, needs to be done carefully and respectfully. I can't just turn up with no explanation – we need to have some conversations and learn to trust each other. We probably need a break before I move back in. And I've thought about living with Noelia, as she was sort of looking for a lodger, but as much as I love her, I don't think I can intrude like that. I might live with Nanna for a while, maybe. I think she'd love it.

But last thing I want to do right now is go from silly and happy with relief to shouting at Dad and everything being awful.

'Chloe! Come and see!' he calls.

'Oh, Dad...'

I go up the stairs. The door to his room is open and there are a few mugs on his floor I can see from here. I'll have to come in and clean.

'Chloe, come on!'

The lights are on, but I can see up the attic stairs and it isn't the blinding white light I remember from when I was in here last. He's gutted and cleared it all.

He's rambling on about doing something with the space, like turning it into a games room, which will never happen. But the weed is gone.

'Why didn't you tell me?' As I climb the ladder I can see even the foil and fans have disappeared. There are no plant pots, it's empty.

'Oh, yeah. Like you were listening. Stubborn as stone....' Dad smiles and shakes his head. I remember how isolated and terrified I've been in the last few weeks; the constant drag of not knowing if I'll pass placement, Karen's sharp smiles and Christopher. His nightly texts have stopped.

'Knew it was mad not to just drag you up here, you must have been thinking it was all still going on. As soon as you got back I emptied it all out and sold the rest. But they know now, it isn't a house where we can grow anything, I swear. And to be honest, it's not a nice scene right now, not like when I was younger. They're all a bit... serious,' he says, looking around at the rafters and plaster board.

I look at him in disbelief.

'But I tried to tell you that!'

'Yeah, well, I know how upset you were when you came back. You looked like Helga when she gets scared, all puffed up but basically just terrified and I realised –'

He thinks for a moment, frowning, his head bowed because of the low roof.

'Your Mum would have wanted me to get through however I could. I don't think she would have been that angry about the smoking bit.' He holds his hands up as I start to protest. 'But scaring you like that. You going to live with some bloke I know nothing about, first Ali out of the house and then you... I remember when you were both babies. And Chloe, when you have your own you'll realise, they're only at home for five minutes and then you turn round and they're gone and you're left thinking, what happened? Where did my girls go? Bud's not cocaine or something, but caring about it so much, growing it, not spending any time with you, it just started to take over.'

'Well,' I say, 'Midwifery and everything else took over for me.'

'But that's a good thing to be doing. Like your Mum. It's right for you to be occupied with uni right now and find your feet as an adult. There'll come a time when you're ready to move out of here properly and maybe this bloke of yours is the right one and you'll settle down with him, or someone else... but you shouldn't have felt forced –'

'Dad. Okay.' It's amazing that he can put it all into words. But they are just words. It doesn't mean he can promise never to cause problems. I step carefully back on the ladder and he climbs down too.

'You're so like your Mum,' he says, and though I know he's always going to be up to something, and I'll have to cope with it when it comes, he's my own familiar Dad again.

Wednesday, 22nd August 2001

This time on a Saturday, especially during the summer break, Christopher might still be in bed. But I have a key. And I did text him last night to let him know I was coming over in the morning.

I'm going along New Walk, the red asphalt lined with long-established sycamores and oaks, which joins Victoria Park to town. It's the long way round but it's fresh and quiet and I want the time to think. I'm in my black skirt and a little light blue top and I've straightened my hair. I woke at 6am – I'm still used to getting up early for placement – but I've waited until eight to start to walk over to Christopher's.

I did fall for him. But it's like a drug, a huge cascade of drugs, and falling in love with the wrong person can happen. I think the whole abortion thing has made me think and feel differently. I'm jumpy and guilt-ridden, but mixed with that I'm calm and resigned. In some ways my feelings towards Christopher are softer because I want to protect him from having to think about what happened. But I'm not sure it's right to keep it from him. I haven't quite decided if I'll tell him, but I think he deserves to know: he deserves to learn from it as much as me.

I let myself in and the flat is quiet. The blue carpet, the orderly kitchen side, a basket of clean washing on the sofa all look odd; I've forgotten what it's like to see them every day. I usually love how smell can bring back memories. I often feel close to Mum when I smell her old shampoo (I've hidden a bottle in the back of the bathroom cupboard) but the lemon air freshener and cleaning products that Christopher uses are just making me sad.

Now I'm here, I'm not quite sure what to do with myself. There are some cups and bowls out and I know he hates his draining board being cluttered so I start putting them away, very slowly and quietly, so I don't wake him if he's still asleep. I don't think I've made enough noise to reach upstairs, but maybe I'm wrong, because I hear the bedroom door open and Christopher walk to the bathroom. He pees loudly and then runs the water to wash his hands.

I hear him come down the stairs and into the kitchen. He's in his yellow towelling dressing gown and has a sleep-crumpled face.

'Morning,' I say.

His eyes widen as he sees me and he makes a yelping noise.

'Sorry, Christopher, I didn't mean to scare you. Hi.'

I'm not sure whether to go over and kiss him on the cheek, but in the end I don't, because he's hovering in the doorway and looking at me like I'm a mirage.

'I knew you'd be in, I was up early... Christopher?'

'You should have told me you were coming,' he says, pulling his dressing gown around himself and retying the knot. His words are coming out fast and high-pitched. 'It's been nearly a month! Jesus Christ, Chloe.'

I'm not offended. I don't blame him, but I don't know how else I could have handled things until I had the space to think. He flaps his hands at me.

'Now's not a good time. You should go. Now.'

'Okay. I'm sorry. I did text to say I was coming over... but I can't leave until we've talked.'

'It's my house!'

'Yeah, but we need to talk. Get a cup of coffee first. You always need coffee at this time in the morning, c'mon.' I wave at the machine.

While he finds a cup and hits the button on the machine I sit on the sofa, wanting some distance between his anger and me. For something to do, I start folding his washing.

'I'll go and put some proper clothes on,' he says, then turns around and sees what I'm doing.

'You don't have to do that, stop doing that!' There's a snarl in his voice. I drop the t-shirt and hold my hands up.

'Okay, okay...' for a second I worry about being alone with him in this mood, with what I have to tell him. But I push the thought away. He might be many things, but I don't think Christopher is violent. But still, I think of the home birth I've just been to, and Simon and Dawn, and I can't help but feel the wrongness of all this.

'You don't need to put proper clothes on. Just... come and sit with me. I really need to tell you some things.'

I pat the sofa beside me, but he backs away. I'm confused by this. I expected anger, frustration, shouting after I told him, but not this tension, like he's going to jump out of his skin, like an angry cat.

'I'm sorry I've been away. I had to go to London. And then Dad... well, I think leaving sorted him out. I think it scared him. But it's all okay now.'

'What, did you take him to rehab or something?'

I laugh, shakily.

'No. I think he just saw how much it was hurting me. Look, this is going to be really hard. I don't know what you're going to think. But we need to talk about it.'

'Are you going to get to the fucking point?'

I look up. I've only heard him swear a handful of times, and it's never been directed at anyone.

'Christopher –'

And then the shower starts running.

'That's Brian,' he says, at once. 'I had a swimming session yesterday. We went out for a drink, that's why I didn't check my phone...'

'Oh,' I say slowly, 'Okay. Where did he sleep?'

'In the spare room.'

'Oh. Right. Maybe we should wait until he's gone? This conversation is a big deal. At least for me.'

He looks furious, 'Are you breaking up with me?'

'No... Christopher, I would never say it like that, I –'

'Chris? Have you got any conditioner?' someone calls down the stairs. It's a woman's voice. I look at Christopher and he stares at me.

'That's Brian's girlfriend, she came round to see him.'

I look at him. I think I recognise the voice. My mouth is dry and dread is spreading through me.

'Chloe, no, come back, you can't just march up there with no warning –'

But I race up the dark stairs to the bathroom, thinking, *I'm going to feel like such an idiot if I'm wrong about this but –*

I knock on the shower door. There's no reply.

'I'm sorry about this, but I'm coming in!'

I push open the door and it's Mia, *fucking Mia*, stood there in a towel, thin and scrawny with a tangle of dark hair and eyeliner running down her wet face.

'Chloe, get out of the bathroom!' She draws herself to her full height and slams the door. I stand there, stunned. She starts shouting, it's muffled and I can hear her moving around, probably getting her clothes on as fast as possible.

I feel ill, uncomprehending, and wonder if she's just come around for homework help or something. I've got this wrong. *Please.*

'I don't know what you expect, it's your fault! You left him on his own and didn't tell him why! Poor guy, he was beside himself last night!'

I stand in the corridor with the image of Mia crashing down around me. I shut my eyes and have a horrible visual of her on top of Christopher.

She bursts out of the door. I can see her dark nipples under her white shirt.

'Chloe! You can't just leave people like that with no reason, they move on, right!?'

I blink at her. She's got a white towel in one hand, the one I used when I was here. She's got foundation on it.

'You don't get it! Like when you were first going out, he loved you but he had to get it somewhere! He was totally loyal once you started doing it, I swear to God, but you can't just make someone stop having sex because you're not up for it! It's hard for him, everyone screws around a little bit, it doesn't mean –'

And that's enough. Whatever else she says doesn't matter. I turn around and go back down the stairs, my heart beating in my ears. I can still hear her shouting and I want to get out of here, I don't want to give her the chance to tell me any more. I think I've got the salient facts.

Downstairs, Christopher has frozen. He looks ashamed, tired and confused and I feel like I'm a lighthouse and he's sliding away from the shore. I remember Dad standing in the attic with weed plants in the background wearing the same expression that Christopher has now.

'Can we talk about this?' he asks.

'No.'

'Chloe, I really think if you got some counselling, if we both went, because I lo –'

'Please don't. I really don't want to hear it.'

'We both have a part to play in this.'

'Well, that might be true.'

My heart is racing. I have no idea what to say. I want to cry, then laugh. Or maybe the other way around. I cross the room to put my trainers back on. I'd usually wear boots or heels with this skirt. I nearly did, so he knew I was making an effort.

I open the front door.

'Don't be here on Monday. I'm coming for my stuff and I'll drop off the key then, too.'

I don't look at him again before I leave.

22

Concealed and Unconcealed

Wednesday, 22nd August 2001, ongoing

I wander down Narborough Road in a daze, no idea where I'm going, past shop tables loaded up with fruit and veg in bright pyramids, with posters for gigs tacked underneath them.

Leaving fast was the best thing I could have done. I'm proud of that. I could have sat around for ages talking with Christopher, shouting and hurting, trying to work out how long it had been going on for. Oh, God. I remember that time his supervisor came around because he couldn't find him on campus. Was that one of them? I have a million questions.

Is this why I knew what to do? Is my brain clever enough to steer me through all this without knowing exactly what was going on, but knowing that I wasn't in the relationship that was being presented?

I'm checking myself over mentally and it's not so bad.

I've been through so much worse with Mum and Dad. The one upside of having my history is that this is small fry. Intense sadness and anger I can cope with; it's the lack of control that I hate so much, where the world is moving under your feet and you might fall. But it looks like I was in control this time. I'll never even have to tell him. I have a wave of elation: I did the right thing.

I walk past the closed South Indian takeaways, quiet and clean with their ugly 1970s decor and paper flowers. The cars rolling past catch the sunlight in their windows and dazzle me. What was he saying about loving me? Can you love someone and still lie to them?

I stop at the Narborough Road bookshop and stare in. There's a copy of Jane Eyre in the window. Jos and I used to love that book, after we studied it in Year 9.

Jos. I get my mobile out of my bag and speed dial her and despite the fact I haven't called in weeks she picks up after a few rings.

'Chloe?'

'Hey,' I say 'Uh. I'm not sure where to start.'

'Oh no, what's wrong?' Her voice is rough and unsteady.

'Jos – are you crying?'

'No.'

'Oh, come on.'

'I might have been earlier,' she says, gulping, 'I… This isn't something for over the phone. But what's up with you?'

'That doesn't sound good. What's up?' I ask again.

There's a silence.

I remember her in the Charlotte, before all of this, before I even started training. I've been meaning to be around more for Jos for over a year and instead I've let us drift.

'Jos. Are you at home?' I say, 'D'you want me to come over?'

'I'm at Hamza's.'

'Oh, right. Shall I come over there, then? Will his parents mind?

'Yes. I mean, no, they won't mind. Yes please. Come over.'

I ask her a few more times, but she won't tell me what's going on. Eventually I hang up. I'm wondering if Hamza or his parents are listening in the background or something. I walk quickly to get to St Margaret's bus station and get the 42 out to Oadby where Hamza's parents have a big house, in a nice area, with lots of rooms. Most of their kids have left by now, but it was always full of their cousins and friends when we were growing up.

I'm still surprised that I seem to be basically okay. I'll tell Jos what happened with Christopher, but I'm not sure I can tell her anything else. We can sort out what's wrong with her though.

I get off the bus and walk a few streets over to Hamza's and when I ring the bell his Dad answers.

'Hello Mr Ibrahim. Is Jos here?'

He's a big man, a school teacher with a wiry black beard and intelligent eyes. I've always been a bit scared of him, but in current circumstances I don't seem to be afraid of anything.

He welcomes me in with his normal formality. The house is clean-smelling, the scent of soap and the barest hint of onions and spice in the background. Everything is so organised: twenty pairs of shoes in a see-through storage unit by the door, arranged by size and type.

A small child with brown eyes fringed with thick lashes pops his head around the kitchen door and giggles at me. He looks like Hamza did when he was young, how I remember him in primary school.

I smile and wave back, but a woman I don't recognise picks the boy up under his arms and takes him further into the house without looking at me. I slip off my shoes and follow Mr Ibrahim past the lounge, which is tiled with concentric blue and white patterns and has huge silver copies of the

Qur'an over the mantel piece.

At the foot of the stairs he says, 'You're needed today. Jos needs her friends.'

I'm mystified.

'You young people. If we don't listen to you then we're fools. I'm sorry,' he says, and then he points me up the stairs and tells me Jos is staying in Hamza's sister's room.

I pad upwards, confused, knock on the door and Jos answers. She's not wearing her headscarf, I suppose because she has privacy in this room. Her hair is long, she's grown it and she looks like the old Jos I remember from childhood and my heart tightens. Her eyes are red and puffy. She's been crying, a lot.

'Jos, what the hell is going on?'

She doesn't answer. I hug her and tell her it's all going to be okay and her fingers press hard into my back. She looks desperate. We arrange ourselves on the bedspread, in Hamza's sister's powder pink room, and I watch her carefully.

She exhales.

'They made me a quilt as soon as they found out. They're trying.'

My heart starts beating faster; this is an old Ibrahim family ritual. Baby clothes and old school uniforms and childhood curtains and other bits of fabric that are full of meaning are cut up into hexagons and stitched together into a patchwork. This is a present the Ibrahim girls get when they're getting married, so they have something to take to their new home. For a moment, I think Hamza and Jos must have eloped.

'Found out what?' I ask.

'I just... give me a second.' She closes her eyes.

'Jos, you're scaring me. Are you ill?'

Her eyes fly open.

'No! Oh sorry, Chloe, it's nothing like that, I swear. It's okay.'

'You're okay?'

'Yes. I will be. I'm just trying to find the words.'

'Thank God.' I feel like weeping. 'Can you tell me? Just get it out in one go.'

'Ha.' She laughs and touches her forehead 'How to say it...'

'Okay. Build up to it then. Tell me about the quilt. This is yours? It's lovely.'

We admired Hamza's sister's patchwork quilt when we were twelve or thirteen. I remember Jos telling me that she'd have one, one day. And here we are.

'They gave me the scraps left over. They'd already started making one for a cousin, they just added to it. They asked Mum for my old baby clothes but she wouldn't give them to them. They did go over there, but she won't really talk. They're not really sure what to do, they're trying to make me feel welcome and they know that supporting me is the right thing. It's my own fault. He's their favourite boy and now I've brought shame on the whole family...'

I can hear small noises, water splashing, the murmur of women's voices in the kitchen.

Jos puts her head in her hands and I suddenly realise what she's trying to tell me.

'Jos. Are you in trouble in *that* way?'

She looks at me with a pleading expression, collapses against the wall behind her and puts one hand on her stomach.

'Oh Jos...' I breathe.

I remember when she was tiny and we were both in primary school. We swapped brightly coloured erasers, bought our first mascara together and whispered about shaving our legs with razors stolen from our Mums. I try to find the right thing to say.

'It's not your fault. What you did... it's only natural, you love each other. And isn't it Hamza's responsibility just as much as yours?'

'Yeah. Well, I think they think I tricked him into it...'

'Jos, what *did* happen? You were so certain you wouldn't.'

'It just got too much.' She looks at me. It occurs to me I'm getting so tired of women crying about things like this. I hardly ever see men cry. Apart from that dad at the home birth. Where do you find men like that?

'We started revising together round his brother's. He works at the school. We'd have these long hours together and we'd just be having a cuddle in front of the TV and it turned into... well, something else. And we didn't do anything that I could have got pregnant from for a really long time. And then we did and it just felt... I was filled up with love for him. I thought Allah wasn't angry.'

She looks at me and her voice stops shaking.

'So what are you going to do?' I ask her.

She shrugs.

'In Islam, we should wait until the baby's born to get married. But we might get married sooner. I think the family want it all sorted and they're being amazing. They want me to keep going with uni and everything.'

'Right... and how are you? How are you coping?'

'I'm alright. You said something had happened, though, is everyone okay? How's your Dad? And Christopher?'

'We don't have to talk about it.'

'I've been thinking about my stuff a lot, lately, believe it or not. We can come back to it. Let's do yours,' she says.

'Ha. Okay. Dad's... he's better. He's sorted himself out. He went through a phase of growing weed in the attic –'

'Of course. Was that why you moved in with Christopher?'

I love how casual she is. Always unflappable when it comes to anything my family does.

'Yeah. Well I had to, I couldn't keep living at home expecting the police to pop round every minute. But it didn't last long. Me moving out gave him a kick up the bum and I'm living back there now.'

Her eyes widen.

'But what about Christopher?'

'Christopher... well, that didn't end so well.'

'End? What d'you mean, end?'

'Well. I had this feeling it wasn't right, even though it was really serious. And I just went around to talk to him today and he's definitely slept with Mia, but probably other girls too.'

'What! Oh my God, that cheating piece of shit... Chloe, are you okay?'

I look at her and smile.

'I will be.'

'Are you trying to be zen or something? He slept with one of your friends, he's scum! Oh, if I spot Mia anywhere... she'd better think about leaving Leicester. Wait until everyone finds out!'

'Yeah. I know. I'm not feeling angry though. Yet. Maybe I will later but I think I'm just relieved. I moved out of Christopher's about a month ago. I just thought I couldn't rely on him. And I was right.'

'Any other surprises for me?'

'That's about it.' *Tell her, tell her.* No. She won't understand. We sit on the bed for a while, holding hands. Then I say,

'Jos, you know... you don't have to... you get to choose. Anything you want. Have you thought about everything? All your options?'

'I know what you're asking,' she says. Anger rises up her throat and into her voice. 'I could never do that. I could never live with myself.'

I watch her get up and put her black hijab back on. She's reflected in the bedroom mirror. She tucks in the black cloth left and right and pats her head to check it's all in place and she looks taller and steadier and more peaceful.

I think of the garden, the raspberry bushes, the ground lit by the August sun. I wrap my arms around myself and draw my knees into my chest.

'Okay, I'll be here for you,' I say. 'Whatever you need. Whatever you want.'

Epilogue

Sunday, 26th August 2001

And finally, during the summer break, there's a day for myself.

There's something so amazing about being unhurried and I wake up slowly. I know how close I was to working frantically through the whole three weeks and as I get up and open my curtains I stand and smile in the warm sunshine.

This morning isn't so different from the Sundays I used to have before midwifery training. I'll make tea and toast and do a bit of cleaning. But back before I got my uni place, I'd always have the thought in the back of my mind about when midwifery might start. I knew it would happen eventually, but it was a constant question on repeat.

And then there's Christopher. Still some stuff to work through there. I can't help but feel that someone more attractive wouldn't have been cheated on, though this isn't my fault. But I'm glad to be free. The bliss of being alone isn't something I'd be experiencing if I was waking up in Christopher's bed.

I wonder how Jos is getting on. When I left her at Hamza's, being looked after by his sister and cousins, she said to me,

'It's okay, I've been blessed. It just shouldn't have happened this way.'

I might never tell her what I chose. Even though it was right, that was only because it was my choice. Her decision is based on what she wants, so that's right too. Same with Sadie.

I smile. Mum would say I was being too serious and to make sure I have some fun. I wish beyond anything I could talk to her; she'd know exactly what to say to put this year in the context of my whole life. And I bet she would have had suggestions regarding Karen, too.

There's so much at stake for me when I'm training. I sometimes wonder if my obsession with this career makes it harder and whether I should learn to distance myself. I'd find it all easier because I wouldn't be fighting, I could just let things go. This is, in part, what Christopher was trying to say.

But despite everything, I know keeping this desire fresh and burning is my only option. I can't turn my passion off. I can't wait to be back on placement again, getting into the women's lives, putting my hands on their bumps to feel their babies, hearing heartbeats. I never thought midwifery would be easy, I never asked it to be. I just wanted to be part of it. Now I have even more feeling to bring with me.

If you enjoyed this book please look out for the next installment of Chloe's training.

The number one thing you can do to help me as a first-time author and the small but awesome independent publisher Pinter & Martin is to leave an honest review of this book online. That way more readers can find it. And I can get on with book two.

Thank you!

Ellie

For updates and midwifery blogging, subscribe to MidwifeDiaries.com

Can't wait for the next installment?
Here is the first chapter of Open my Eyes, that I may see
marvellous things *by Alice Allan, which you may also like...*

The doctors' café of St George's Hospital smells of cinnamon tea and mango juice, coffee and cardamom. The sweet, spicy scents mingle with the earthier smell of the old building. The patients' various odours of poverty and disease don't permeate here.

Chatter and laughter echo off the tiled walls. The sounds are joined by the clinking of cups and the clang of oxygen cylinders being delivered. Sitting here, in my midwife's scrubs, red-brown skin, cap over my braided hair, I fit into the medical crowd. Here, I am camouflaged as I drink my coffee. Surrounded by all these East Africans, I could pass for one of them. But I know better. I am an interloper. Thirty-three years in England makes me more English than Ethiopian.

My birth mother's here, in Ethiopia, somewhere, unless she is already dead, which is highly likely. Everyone said I'd go looking for her. When I went off to do my voluntary service overseas, even my adoptive mum, June, thought she would lose me to another woman, and since Dad died I'm all the family she has. She needn't have worried. I proved them wrong. Call it stubborn, but I just don't see the point of looking. I'm here in Addis Ababa to work and learn; to build up professional experience so I can say that I 'walked the walk'. Anyway, I don't need to find her; I know her quite well enough already.

I see her in the faces of the young women on the ward who turn their gaze away from their newborns. Those women are wet coals, damp wood; with them the radiance, the fire of new motherhood does not catch. Perhaps inside those blank bodies they are screaming as they pack their few belongings, avert their eyes from their mouthing babies and walk away. To the observer they seem cold, indifferent. They are hard to forgive. But the other midwives have sometimes shown me the tokens that the mothers leave behind; small wooden crosses, a plastic flower, a piece of red string. Then I forgive them. My birth mother left me no such memento.

Ah, well. Better drink up. My shift's about to start. I drain my coffee cup to the sweet, gritty dregs.

There are nine flights of dusty, dirt-speckled concrete steps to climb to reach the labour ward. Three flights for every month I've got left in Ethiopia. Of course, I'll be doing pretty much the same job when I get back to the UK, but things are more raw here, there's more at stake, and it hurts to think of leaving. I sigh, pausing on a landing. I'm thirty-six. My work is my life. I've been a midwife so long that most of the time I do it without thinking about it. Capable, tidy, efficient. Good in a crisis, that's me. But just sometimes... that look of shocked wonder when a mother meets her child's eyes for the first time gets me when I least expect it. The new dawn of innocence and all that. I know it's just an illusion. Life's destined to disappoint. But it's an illusion that keeps me going. I keep climbing.

The labour ward is cool, the dingy corridor lit by a flickering fluorescent tube. In the tiny office, I read through the notes of the new admissions to see who's arrived, and then check who's been discharged. Through the glass I scan the patients, putting faces to names. There's a skinny girl in bed three who has a scar that pulls the centre of one eye downwards, like an exaggerated teardrop. Her dark face is closed and unreadable. She must be terrified, poor thing. I can't find her notes, but the head midwife updates me.

"She came in this morning. They found her, collapsed outside the hospital. She's thirty-four weeks' gestation but labour has already started."

"That's early, especially since she's malnourished. The baby will be small."

"We are trying to slow it down. Perhaps with bed rest birth can be delayed. But she may lose the child."

"What's her name?"

"She won't give us her name. She says she's eighteen, but I don't believe it. Look at her... she's so small. She says she's from Merkato but her accent is from the country. She's probably just been sleeping in the market since she got to Addis."

The girl replies to questions monosyllabically, in an almost inaudible mutter, but I already know her story. One of seven or eight siblings, probably, not counting the ones who died in childhood. Her family scrape a living on some hillside, far from any main road. She'll have been taken from school when she was twelve to help at home with the cooking and the younger children, then at fifteen, to avoid a long-arranged marriage to an older man, she'll have run away to Addis, set on becoming a housemaid, with a uniform and a little box room to call her own. But people will have taken her shy country ways for sullenness, wrinkled their noses at the rancid smell of the *kebe* butter she dressed her hair in. She'll have been ruled out of work because she didn't know how to use an iron or a vacuum cleaner. Hungry, she'll have begged in the street, unable to return. One night, maybe for many nights, she'll have taken coins from a man who filled her belly in more ways than one.

The midwife interrogates her.

"Have you been eating well? Did you have any check-ups? You're lucky you're not HIV positive," she says, scanning her blood test results. "Next time use a condom."

The girl turns her face away at the insensitive suggestion. To speak of such things is shameful; besides, men will pay more for not having to wear one and rough up girls who insist.

"The baby is small," says the midwife. "We may not be able to stop it coming."

I pat her arm. We give her steroids to mature the baby's lungs and tell her to rest.

Half an hour later, though, she tries to stand to go to the toilet and her waters break. She begins to contract more strongly and there is no way now to prevent labour.

I wheel her to the delivery room. While we wait for the obstetrician, I put on gloves and ease her stiff legs apart. I move two fingers inside her, feeling for the soft ring of her cervix; she gasps with pain. She is six centimetres dilated. It won't be long before she is ready to deliver.

"Baby is coming," I tell her in my clumsy Amharic. I wish I knew more words so I could comfort her. Instead I make do with rolling her onto her side and massaging her back with the heel of my hand. The minutes pass. The doctor does not come, but soon the baby will.

The pains come close together now; she does not cry out, but writhes, her arms above her head, gripping the bars of the metal bed. I see the beads of sweat on her top lip. Finally, the obstetrician sweeps in, and five students, all men, troop in with her.

I brief the doctor in English. The students look bored by the girl's labouring. Probably they are embarrassed. One checks his mobile, another yawns and looks out of the window at the swaying tops of the cypress trees. The girl closes her eyes, as if she could pretend the shame and pain away. The doctor makes her put her feet onto boards that stick out from the bottom of the bed; she must hoick her knees up to tighten the pressure in her belly and present her private parts for delivery. I hold her hand; with each strong contraction, she grips it tightly.

The doctor examines her again. She tuts loudly.

"When did they cut you?" she scolds, running her gloved thumb over the scarred lump of the girl's excised clitoris. "They shouldn't cut you. It's illegal. It's not allowed any more, do you hear? If you have a female baby and you cut her, you will be taken to prison. Do you understand?"

She whimpers in understanding. I squeeze her arm tight. It was hardly her fault. She was probably only a baby herself.

Another contraction comes, a strong one that transforms her belly into a hard egg. She writhes and hunches, pushing down with her feet onto the boards.

"This baby won't come," says the doctor cursorily. "I will have to cut you. You need an episiotomy."

The young woman nods blankly. As the obstetrician is reaching for her surgical scissors I lay my hand on her shoulder to stop her, smiling, but not with my eyes.

"You don't need to do that," I caution.

She draws herself up, offended, but I hold my ground. Does she not see the irony of this other kind of cutting? She won't add injury to insult on my watch. Her hand hovers over the scissors before moving away.

"You can try to push," she tells the girl.

So the girl strains, grunting. Pauses. Turns to me, round-eyed.

"It hurts," she says, dismayed. Another contraction comes, a strong one, and with just one more push the baby finally slides out of her.

The baby is tiny and blue and female. It is covered in whitish vernix and it doesn't breathe to start with. We work quickly to resuscitate it with a mask and bag. Its flaccid body twitches into life but its breathing is erratic, so it is bundled up in blankets and taken to the intensive care unit for monitoring. I am left with the girl. I would rather they had kept the baby with its mother; given that little scrap a few minutes of pleasure.

After they've washed her down, and taped a precious sanitary pad onto her bare skin to catch the worst of the bleeding (like many of the women I've seen come in, she doesn't own a pair of knickers), she tells me her name. It is T'irunesh. It means 'you are good'. She can't be much more than sixteen. She doesn't ask me how the baby is.

"Does the baby have a father?" I ask her.

She keeps turning her face away as if it will make these questions go away. I suddenly feel exasperated by her.

"You are a mother now. How you are going to look after this baby?" I ask impatiently.

The girl turns to me then with a look of astonishment that makes me shut my mouth with a snap; I see that it has never once occurred to her that she would keep the baby. For a few seconds, I am face-to-face with my mother on the day she had me.

Open my Eyes, that I may see marvellous things *by Alice Allan is published by Pinter & Martin and available from all good bookshops, online retailers, pinterandmartin.com and as an ebook*